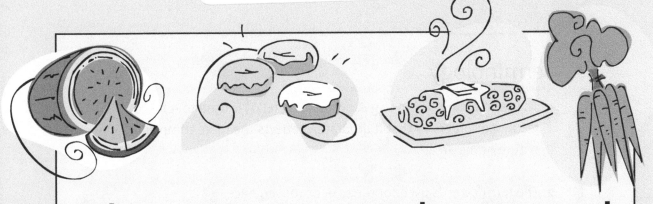

The Fun with Food Programme

Therapeutic intervention for children with aversion to oral feeding

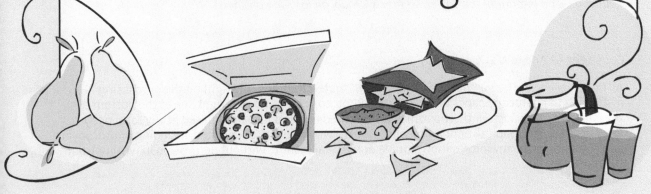

Edited by Arlene McCurtin

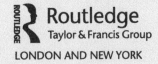

Routledge
Taylor & Francis Group

LONDON AND NEW YORK

Terminology

1 The term eating & drinking & swallowing (EDS) is used to refer to feeding disorders so that it accurately reflects the more complex nature of the area.

2 The term 'carer' is used for the sake of convenience.

3 The term 'clinician' is used in place of 'therapist' to reflect all members of the interdisciplinary team.

4 For the purpose of clarity alone, 'he' is used to refer to clients.

For Aisling, David, Ciara, Andrew and Luke

First published 2007 by Speechmark Publishing Ltd.

Published 2017 by Routledge
2 Park Square, Milton Park, Abingdon, Oxon OX14 4RN
711 Third Avenue, New York, NY 10017, USA

Routledge is an imprint of the Taylor & Francis Group, an informa business

British Library Cataloguing in Publication Data
McCurtin, Arlene
 The fun with food programme
 1. Eating disorders in children – Treatment
 I. Title
 618.9'2852606

ISBN-13: 9780863885662 (pbk)

Contents

List of Tables

Foreword

The Fun with Food programme originated from a need to develop more efficient and more effective services for children with disabilities who had an aversion to oral feeding. As its originator, I worked within an interdisciplinary team, all of whose members were committed to creating improved options both for the children and their carers, and for the clinicians involved in offering those services.

In presenting this material the intention is that clinicians will adapt it to both the resources at their disposal and to the needs of the clients.

I hope you will find applications for your practice.

Arlene McCurtin

Acknowledgements

Thanks to all the clinicians who came on board enthusiastically with the Fun with Food programme when it was originally proposed, who helped to develop and sustain it, and who shared their skills. Thanks also to the children and their families who committed themselves to the programme in its early days.

Contributors

Marie Kennedy, *Dietetics Manager, Central Remedial Clinic, Dublin*
Jeni Malone, *Senior Occupational Therapist, Central Remedial Clinic, Dublin*
Arlene McCurtin, *Lecturer, Clinical Therapies, University of Limerick, Limerick*
Ger McGuirk, *Senior Dietitian, Central Remedial Clinic, Dublin*
Trish Morrison, *Senior Speech & Language Therapist, Central Remedial Clinic, Dublin*
Damhnait Ní Mhurchú, *Senior Speech & Language Therapist, Central Remedial Clinic, Waterford*
Petro Van Deventer, *Senior Speech & Language Therapist, South Africa*

Contributions are acknowledged. Those not done so are the work of the main contributor and editor, Arlene McCurtin.

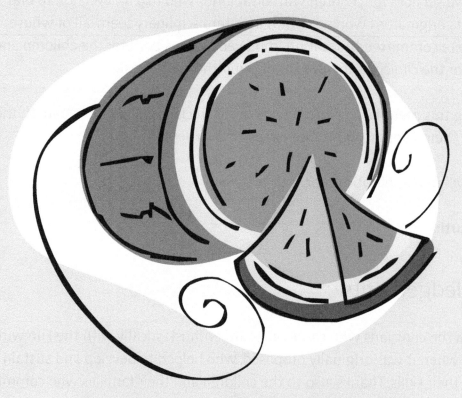

Introduction

Healthy eating and drinking are at the core of our development. Aversion to oral eating, for whatever reason, compromises a child's development. In severe cases it can have a profound effect, mostly with respect to nutrition and hydration, but it also puts children at risk of developing intellectual and educational problems. As mealtimes are occasions to provide social, communication and interaction opportunities, eating & drinking & swallowing (hereafter referred to as EDS) aversion may also cause significant carer anxiety and affect child–carer and peer relationships. It is therefore important, not just for the child's nutritional status, development and general health but also for the success of the child–carer relationship, to focus intervention in this area. Furthermore, it is largely agreed that children with medically based problems are at risk of additional behavioural problems, unless the original problems are resolved quickly (Christophen & Hall 1978; Linscheid 1978; Palmer & Horn 1978).

What is the Fun with Food programme?

The Fun with Food programme provides an option for the treatment of selective and total aversive oral eaters. It can be adapted by the clinician to provide one-to-one treatment where resources and circumstances dictate. However, it is strongly recommended that any adaptation have a carer group as a core component. Additionally, videotaping is utilised as an integral part of the Fun with Food approach to develop carer skills, and the clinician should access this facility if possible.

Essentially, the Fun with Food approach to aversive oral eating is multicomponent and multidisciplinary, with emphasis placed on carer training. This facilitates the development of understanding of EDS aversion, generalisation of skills and a hands-on approach to treatment.

The programme is dominated by the five main stages outlined in Table 1 on page 2.

Table 1: Outline of the Fun with Food approach to aversive EDS treatment

Stage	Aim
1. Assessment	■ Obtain baseline of EDS skills ■ Identify specific problem areas ■ Identify presence or absence of EDS aversion ■ Determine suitability for programme ■ Determine suitability for pre-feeding component of programme
2. Food for Thought: Carer training	■ Develop understanding of EDS generally ■ Carer empowerment ■ Develop readiness for intervention stages of programme ■ Access to peer support
3. Fun before Food: Pre-feeding intervention	■ Develop those skills which may form the support structure for improvement in EDS skills (oral motor function, sensory skills, food play)
4. EDS: Eating & drinking & swallowing intervention	■ EDS immersion to facilitate both carer and child skill development generally ■ Develop food approach skills in child ■ Develop interaction and management skills in carer ■ Extend range of tastes and textures taken ■ Where appropriate move, decrease or eliminate dependence on tube feeding for nutrition ■ Increase oral intake for nutritional purposes
5. More Food: Review Days	■ Monitor progress ■ Develop EDS skills further ■ Continue with group support system

Who is the Fun with Food programme for?

The programme was originally designed to develop more efficient and effective services for groups of children with disabilities who presented with aversion to oral eating. However, it is by nature adaptable to both client groups and contexts such as special schools and child development centres. Thus far it has been used to treat individuals with:

■ physical disabilities
■ learning disabilities
■ autism

- Down syndrome
- sensory processing disorders
- complex medical histories but no overt diagnoses.

Clinicians are encouraged to adapt the programme to their own and client needs and this includes one-to-one intervention. The criteria typically used for inclusion in the programme are as follows:

1 *Presence of aversion* to oral eating, drinking and swallowing; that is, aversion to all or some aspects of oral eating, from taking nothing orally to oral selectivity such as lump refusal. Aversion is present when it constitutes refusal outside norms and is not due to pathology, although it may have its roots in a medical condition.
2 *Medical stability.* Children with medical issues are not excluded but they must be medically able to undertake an EDS programme, particularly with regard to neurological and respiratory conditions. Children who are aspirators can be included in the programme; however, use of 'unsafe' consistencies would be avoided until clinicians are confident of the child's oral motor and swallow functions.
3 *Nutritional stability.* Children must be nutritionally stable and able to afford to lose some weight as determined by a dietitian.
4 *Carer commitment.* Carers should attend for the duration of the course. Where possible, two carers should be in attendance.
5 *Group fit* is the best match of individuals based on characteristics such as degree of aversion, physical ability, presence of tube feeding and so on. Group homogeneity may facilitate successful outcomes. Depending on the group and resources, the clinician may want to match for selective or total aversive oral eaters.

Clinicians can also use individual programme elements instead of the whole programme; for example, the Fun before Food pre-feeding programme may be used with a child who is not yet ready for oral feeding, or the EDS programme may be suitable for a child who has no pre-feeding issues. The intention with this book is to provide guidelines for aversive EDS treatment, and not dictate a 'one solution fits all' philosophy.

The programme is constructed to meet the needs of a variety of age groups and populations as can be seen in Table 2 below, which reflects the characteristics of one group.

Table 2: Sample of actual group on the Fun with Food programme

Characteristic	Breakdown
Gender	6 boys, 2 girls
Diagnoses	3 syndromes, 2 physical disability, 2 learning disability, 1 no diagnosis
Aversion	3 totals, 5 selectives
Chronological age	4.02–9.01 years (mean 5.0) – does not reflect developmental age
Nutritional status	None underweight
Tube feeding	4 PEG (gastrostomy) fed at time of commencement, 3 of whom had nil oral intake 6 with a history of naso-gastric feeding
Use of supplements	2 on supplements at time of commencement of programme
Oral motor skills	4 presented with moderate oral motor dysfunction 2 presented with normal oral motor function 2 refused to co-operate on assessment
Sensory skills	6 of 8 demonstrated sensory processing problems
Aspiration status	2 aspirators based on videofluroscopy studies 1 at-risk aspirator based on videofluroscopy study
Gastro-oesophageal reflux	4 diagnosed with gastro-oesophageal reflux 3 had fundoplications with 1 further recommendation for same

What professionals are involved?

The programme developed from an understanding of the importance of interdisciplinary working in treating EDS disorders. Core personnel are:

- speech & language therapist
- dietitian
- occupational therapist.

Resources permitting, the following disciplines would also be part of the team:

- counsellor (social worker or clinical psychologist)
- paediatrician.

A co-ordinator (typically the speech & language therapist) runs the programme and utilises professional staff to lead various sessions or lectures, or elements of the programme; for example, a psychologist or social worker would run the Carer Support sessions.

The aims of the Fun with Food programme

In treating children with aversion to oral eating, the programme achieves its aims in three main ways:

1 **Support and peer motivation**
   The programme provides carers with opportunities to share ideas, issues and concerns with other carers who are in a similar situation. It also provides support to children through carers, clinicians and peers.

2 **Education**
   The programme helps carers and children develop a broader understanding of EDS skills and issues.

3 **Application**
   The programme provides repeated opportunities for carers and children to practise strategies under guidance and in a structured environment, with the overall intention of increasing oral nutritional intake and developing the range of oral tastes and textures relative to the child's pre-programme performance.

   Some individuals, however, may start with 'non-food' goals, including building up confidence and pleasure around eating, and reducing stress associated with eating.

The core principles of the Fun with Food programme

The core principles underpinning the Fun with Food programme are listed below.

1 Intervention is interdisciplinary

> Feeding problems are not a specific entity but rather are the result of a cluster of related medical, environmental, nutritional and social variables. *(Babbit et al, 1994)*

Oral feeding aversion can vary from simple selectivity (limited repertoire), that is, avoidance of certain foods, to total aversion, that is, zero oral intake. It can be solely about behavioural issues, or originate from a multiplicity of causes, for example, sensory processing, oral motor and medical issues. EDS problems are typically complex and require the skills of a number of different clinicians in order to meet the needs of children and their carers effectively. For example, dietitians enable speech & language therapists to work on EDS aggressively by monitoring weight and ensuring nutritional needs are met. Previously, in the Fun with Food programme, we have utilised the skills of speech & language therapists, dietitians, occupational therapists, psychologists, social workers and paediatricians. Onward referrals to counsellors, radiologists and gastro-enterologists are also made as required.

2 Intervention is intensive
Provision of treatment on an intensive basis gives those receiving treatment more opportunities to develop and carry over skills in a supportive environment. Given the multiple issues surrounding EDS problems, constant revisiting of goals, reconfirmation of principles and numerous opportunities to take part in activities over an intensive period increase the chances of success.

3 EDS immersion
Both children and their carers require repeated opportunities to develop their management and EDS skills in a supported environment. This can be done effectively in an intensive context. Within such a context there are many opportunities to re-evaluate and reset goals, to model EDS skills, to practise interaction skills, to set boundaries and also to try non-preferred foods. Additionally, the praise potential for achieving goals increases significantly in an intensive environment, which can be highly motivating for children.

4 Focus on carer empowerment

Carers and clinicians need to work collaboratively, in partnership and in an open manner if they are to meet the needs of children with EDS aversion effectively. The role of the clinician is to guide and provide the benefit of their clinical experience; however, it is the skills of the carer that will in the end effectively determine the outcome. The whole approach of Fun with Food is carer involvement and carer-led goal setting. In the initial stages of treatment, carers typically require facilitation towards this end as they have often lost direction and confidence in themselves through the 'failure' of their child's oral EDS skills. Carers have usually tried numerous techniques to get their child to eat and end up losing focus and the ability to interpret what works and what does not. They may require remotivation and help in regaining their skills. Developing carer analytical skills through a variety of activities, including videotaping, will make a difference in long-term carry-over.

Understanding the ongoing role carers and not clinicians play in ensuring successful outcomes means providing carers with intensive support through sessions, in carer-to-carer contact, in carer-to-key worker contact and in dedicated carer support groups. No matter how understanding a clinician may be, understanding from a peer in the same situation is of more significant value to a carer.

To facilitate successful partnerships, the clinician is required to share all information and knowledge with carers, which includes written copies of goals, notes, reports and so on. This helps to ensure that decision making is as informed as possible. Informed carers are active carers.

5 Support development of EDS skills through focus on pre-feeding skills

Not all children require this element of the programme; however, for those who do, it can be pivotal in gradually introducing them to food in a non-threatening way. Fun before Food can be run approximately two weeks prior to the main programme in order to give time for carry-over and further development of skills in the areas of sensory processing, oral motor awareness and function, food play, nutrition and normalising responses to food. Fun before Food provides the foundation skills for oral feeding, develops readiness for EDS and facilitates the development of a positive attitude to EDS.

6 Teaching goal-setting skills

Teaching carers to set graded goals facilitates problem definition and treatment planning. Carers' analytical skills are developed through teaching goal setting and constant revisiting of EDS goals and programme aims at defined points: before the course, at each eating and drinking session, at the end of the EDS programme, at each More Food Review Day and so on. Furthermore, both carer and staff programme aims are rated by carers at end of the EDS week, and carer goals for eating are rated after each EDS activity.

Encouraging short- rather than long-term thinking, and teaching carers to break down larger goals into small graded steps based on the child's abilities and performance, are at the cornerstone of intervention. For example, a carer may say 'I want my child to eat'. If the carer continues to think of this as the primary goal, then failure is likely. Instead, carers are encouraged to break down goals, to think about how to achieve their aim in small steps. This may be 'Today at session 1, Johnny will lick a spoon with yoghurt on it, once'. While such an approach can be slow and frustrating for some carers, the long-term outcome of taking expectations and making them achievable for the child by grading them gives carers a concrete point from which to move forward. This creates a 'can do' approach and the expectation of achievement.

7 Reduction of tube feed dependence

Of equal importance to developing oral EDS skills is the necessity to fade tube dependence for nutritional purposes. This is partly to create an appetite. However, in a child who has a history of tube feeding and no real understanding of appetite, hunger or the oral–stomach relationship, simply making a child hungry will not ensure success. Such children require an all-encompassing approach to EDS skills development.

8 Positive thinking

Even if there is a pathological reason for EDS problems, such as the presence of gastro-oesophageal reflux or oral motor dysfunction, when this is managed it does not prevent moving ahead with EDS development. The leap of faith required literally reflects the carer's uptake of the programme, and trust in the skills of the clinician to guide them. Children will then respond to a carer's can-do attitude. Clinicians should facilitate this by providing a supportive and logical environment.

9 Encourage autonomy and independence

Where a child is physically able, the independent feeding should be fostered. Some children may continue to manipulate their carers or search for comfort by attempting to set their own rules, for example, the carer must feed the child even though he is physically able, or the child wants to sit on the carer's lap. Provide the child with a sense of autonomy, and the carers with a sense of freedom. Use of choices is sometimes appropriate, sometimes not. Independence always is.

10 Maintain neutrality in the eating and drinking interaction

Carers are taught to remove all attention from the process, to maintain automaticity in their interaction. This ensures two main things: they do not get 'caught up' in the interaction with the child emotionally and do not end up adjusting goals inappropriately, and the child learns to understand goals, boundaries and expectations.

How the book is structured

The first chapter provides a definition of EDS aversion, and considers the relevance of Fun with Food to an evidence-based approach to its treatment. Thereafter, there are five stages to the programme and each section is given its own chapter:

- **Assessing the child** (Chapter 2)
- **Food for Thought: The carer programme** (Chapter 3)
- **Fun before Food: The pre-feeding programme** (Chapter 4)
- **Fun before Food: The Eating & Drinking & Swallowing (EDS) programme** (Chapter 5)
- **More Food Review Days** (Chapter 6).

At the end of each chapter are photocopiable forms and samples which can be used by clinicians for their own intervention programmes. The photocopiable appendices at the back of the book contain timetables, reports and sample letters.

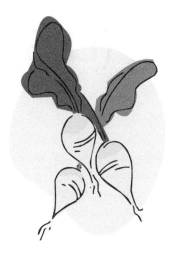

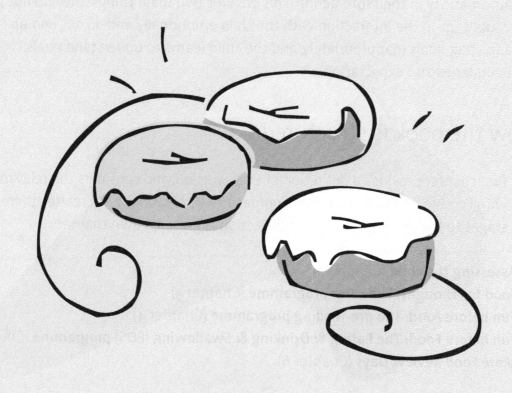

Chapter 1
Eating & Drinking & Swallowing (EDS) Aversion

How is aversion defined?

Typically, aversion to oral eating & drinking & swallowing (EDS) is defined by the child's excessive or extreme and consistently negative reaction to requests to eat and/or drink either any oral foods or such a significant number of oral foods that the range of their intake would not support adequate nutrition on its own (in the case of tastes), or does not reflect their peers' eating and drinking development (as in the case of textures). It is important to remember that all children and adults have food dislikes and this reflects normal behaviour. It becomes aversive when an impact or potential impact on the child's health and/or nutrition results.

The definitions in this programme are shown in Table 3.

Table 3: Definition of aversion

Total aversion	No oral intake of either liquids or solids, resulting in tube dependency for all nutritional requirements.
Selective aversion	Reflects a limited repertoire of intake with regard to tastes or textures, or both.

Harris (2000) provides a more comprehensive definition of aversive eating behaviour, the main ones of which are identified in Table 4 (overleaf).

Harris also discusses oral motor dysfunction and its possible impact as a contributor to aversion to oral EDS. This can be especially relevant when working with children with disabilities who are prone to oral motor problems. It may be an isolated factor or one of many factors contributing to eating problems in this group. A retrospective unpublished study by McCurtin, Kennedy and Kelly of children with intellectual, physical and multiple disabilities identified gastro-oesophageal reflux and a history of naso-gastric tube feeding as significant in their association with EDS aversion. Gestational feeding readiness, and disability (intellectual disability being the most likely to be associated with EDS aversion) were also significant predictors. However, oral motor function and malnutrition were not found to be particularly associated with, or predictive of, aversion in these populations.

The interdisciplinary approach of the programme acknowledges the possibility that aversion may be due not to one single factor but perhaps multiple aetiologies that are interlinked and difficult to distinguish. See Table 5 for some discussion of the literature.

Table 4: Definitions of aversion to oral feeding, based on Harris

Category	Type/Aetiology	Example
Appetite regulation	Impairment of regulation	Russell-Silver syndrome, growth hormone dysfunction.
	Organic factors	Organic factors inhibit good regulation Major: For example, major organ dysfunction Minor: For example, constipation, anaemia.
	Late development of regulation	For example, sleepy infants with poor appetite.
	Aversive factors	Aversion overrides regulation. The following factors will predict food refusal and weight loss: force-feeding, coaxing, coercion and mealtime tension, presentation of disliked food or inappropriate textures.
	Supplementary feeding	If a child is gaining calories from other sources, they may not have appetite if their growth needs are being met.
Food acceptance	'Fussy eater' Idiosyncratic refusal of foods or group of foods, or the refusal on one day but not on the next.	Occurs frequently in 2-year-old children Can be related to past history of vomiting or gastro-intestinal pain Is related to child temperament.
	Adherence to a limited range of foods A fear reaction to any but a few accepted foods, contamination fears, and a marked neophobic response to new foods.	A function of the late introduction of solid foods Linked to problems with 'threshold' or sensory receptivity. Often seen in children within the autistic spectrum disorder. Possibly linked to an inability to make generalisations about food in the early years.

Table 5: Factors associated with EDS aversion

Gastro-oesophageal reflux (GOR)

Up to 75% of children have been shown to have GOR in some studies (Abrahams & Burkitt, 1970; Sondheimer & Morris, 1979; Reyes et al, 1993), with a variable incidence range (15–75%) reported in neurologically impaired children (Rice et al, 1991; Wesley et al, 1993; Rempel et al, 1998). It has been noted that GOR has often been overlooked in children with disabilities because of their communication difficulties (Sullivan & Rosenbloom, 1996). Some authors feel that GOR is a self-limited disorder, with 60–85% of patients having a 'gradual resolution' by 18 months of age (Ferry et al, 1983); however, GOR may be a significant factor in aversion to oral feeding for a number of reasons. Symptoms of GOR as described in the literature include: oesophagitis (Wolf & Glass, 1992); excessive irritability, abnormal posturing, growth failure and malnutrition (Ferry et al, 1983); respiratory problems, post-swallow aspiration and delayed gastric emptying (Sullivan & Rosenbloom, 1996); dysphagia (Gadenstatter et al, 1999); malnutrition (Reilly, 1993); association of feeding with pain, discomfort and reduction in the desire to eat (Wolf & Glass, 1992; Reilly, 1993); fewer adaptive skills and readiness for solids, food refusal, food loss, difficult feeders (Mathisen et al, 1999); food aversion (Byrne et al, 1982).

Naso-gastric feeding (NG)

NG feeding is surrounded by aversive elements particularly in infants who are obligatory nose breathers (Erenberg & Nowak, 1984). Complications from NG feeding can explain why it is recommended for short-term use only, and the literature reports on a variety of these, including: food refusal (Byrne et al, 1982; Moore & Greene, 1985; Patrick et al, 1986; Reilly, 1993; Mathisen et al, 1999); slowed swallowing (Huggins et al, 1999); persistent eating difficulties, panic attacks (Dello Strologo et al, 1997); adverse effects on the development of oral skills (Carroll & Reilly, 1996); negative responses to other oral stimuli; ongoing stimulus for the gag reflex even when the tube is not present, in babies (Wolf & Glass, 1992); deprivation of opportunities to taste (Bayer et al, 1983); interference with the association of eating as a pleasurable experience (Handen et al, 1986); greater risk of pulmonary aspiration and pneumonia inherent on recurrent removal and resiting of the tube (Norton et al, 1996); less vigorous sucking in infants and less volume taken with the tube (Shiao et al, 1995); gastrointestinal, mechanical and metabolic complications (Cataldi-Betcher et al, 1983); altered breathing patterns from nasal obstruction (Erenberg & Nowak, 1984); nasal and pharyngeal irritation (Dobie, 1978); reflux and oesophagitis (Shellato & Malt, 1985); increased mucus production (Benda, 1979). Ferry et al (1983) found that poor-response NG feeding was associated with other medical problems such as chronic pulmonary disease, malabsorption, cerebral palsy and laryngomalacia. As more sensory nerve fibres are present in the mouth than in any other part of the body, the implications for prolonged NG feeding are significant (Nelson & Benabib, 1991).

Table 5: *continued*

Disability

Estimates for EDS problems as high as 80–85% (Stallings et al, 1993; Perske et al, 1997) have been obtained for learning and physically disabled children with a range of 19–61% for learning-disabled individuals (Jones, 1982) and of approximately 40–50% for children with cerebral palsy (Reilly, 1993). Boyle (1991) comments that the presence of cognitive and sensory deficits may compound feeding problems in disabled children, while Carroll & Reilly (1996) note that these sensory deficits in children with cerebral palsy can lead to resistance to oral activities. Other complicating issues include significantly longer mealtimes required for children with cerebral palsy (Gisel & Patrick, 1998), and a high proportion of mothers of children with cerebral palsy do not enjoy mealtimes, with decreased verbal interaction during meals (Reilly & Skuse, 1992). Deficient communication skills in the child with severe disabilities can also complicate the feeding problem (Boyle, 1991), which can lead to fewer choices being offered (Wolf & Glass, 1992), and the development of manipulative behaviours and frustration. Children who may otherwise be unable to assert themselves will often use mealtimes for this purpose (Winstock, 1994). Parents of a disabled child often experience anxiety and guilt and may overcompensate by being either too strict or too lax (Palmer & Horn, 1978). Also, the risk of aspiration may be increased. A child who has aspirated food into the trachea may panic, protecting the airway by refusing food (Blackman, 1998), especially if they have limited communication skills and control over the process. This also holds true for individuals suffering discomfort or pain from conditions such as oesophagitis and GOR, particularly when they go unrecognised and untreated.

Gestational feeding readiness

Early feeding behaviour is considered a sensitive indicator of central nervous system integrity in neonates (Brazleton, 1979; Casear et al, 1982) and it is well documented that the earlier the gestation the higher the incidence of long-term physical and developmental effects (Cooke, 1994; Morell, 1994). It is commonly held that gestation below around 33 weeks means that the infant is not ready for oral feeding. Estimates include 32/34 weeks (Neal, 1995), 33/34 weeks (Casear et al, 1982), 34/35 weeks (Case Smith et al, 1989), >32 weeks and a birth weight below 1,500g (Benda, 1979). It may be that infants born before they are neurologically equipped for oral feeding have higher chances of being aversive than those born after this stage. Maladaptive feeding behaviours may be the result of a number of factors including the inability to co-ordinate sucking, swallowing and breathing, the absence of cough and gag reflexes, delayed gastric emptying and slow motility (Hancock, 1995). 'Overzealous' attempts to feed a premature infant may increase the likelihood of aspiration or necrotising enterocolitis, and an 'overly conservative approach' could contribute to malnutrition (Benda, 1979).

Table 5: *continued*

Malnutrition
Inadequate nutrition is a recognised complication of children with cerebral palsy (Bax, 1989; Mathisen et al, 1999) and children with severe emotional disturbances and mental retardation (Riordan et al, 1980). Energy intake is more critical for patients with severe disabilities because of their inability to clearly communicate hunger and satiety (Stallings et al, 1993). Luiselli (1989) states that the primary outcome of feeding aversion is chronic malnourishment. Previously, malnutrition was seen as an expected part of the disability (Patrick et al, 1986). Bax's (1989) study of 100 severely disabled young people found that 70% were underweight and 40% of the subjects had major feeding problems. In a study of 90 individuals with cerebral palsy it was found that 46% were undernourished and that those undernourished subjects had lower feeding competence scores compared with adequately nourished subjects (Troughton & Hill, 2001). Reduced caloric intake can be due to oral motor dysfunction, poor dentition, behaviour disturbances or early satiety (Palmer & Horn, 1978).

Oral motor dysfunction (OMD)
OMD is common in individuals with neurological impairment (Ottenbacher et al, 1983; Reilly et al, 1996), especially in cases of severe physical disability (Luiselli, 1989) and the physical distress sometimes associated with feeding (eg gagging) 'establishes the feeding situation as an extremely aversive event'. Children with cerebral palsy may take 2–12 times longer to eat (Gisel & Patrick, 1998) due to their OMD, and prolonged mealtimes resulting from it may result in aversion to oral feeding. A link between the severity of OMD and poor growth has been proposed by a number of researchers (Krick & VanDuyn, 1984; Shapiro et al, 1986; Thomessen et al, 1991). Krick & VanDuyn (1984) showed that children with cerebral palsy and OMD were found to be significantly thinner by age and height than their age- and sex-matched counterparts with cerebral palsy but no oral motor impairment.

Evidence

A move towards evidence-based practice in clinical therapies means that we must address the efficacy of introducing any new treatment model to practising clinicians. Issues which must be considered in providing evidence in treatment of disabilities include:

- The heterogeneous nature of the populations – the diversity in type, aetiology and severity. Variability is one of the cornerstones of disability.
- Co-morbidities, which can include growth retardation, learning disability, seizure disorders, visual and auditory disorders, and communication impairments.

- Multiple interacting variables, for example oral motor dysfunction, motor disability, sensory processing dysfunction.
- Longevity. Due to medical and pharmaceutical advances, children with disabilities are now living longer and the whole foundation upon which we base our evidence is changing continuously.
- The infancy of EDS research in general, particularly with regard to paediatrics and interdisciplinary working.
- The typically short-term nature of studies, which may not sit particularly well with the typically long-term nature of intervention with disabled populations.
- Interdisciplinary teamwork. Approaching EDS from multiple points given the nature of disability is essential, but there has been minimal research from this viewpoint.

The Fun with Food approach attempts to address some of these issues as follows:

- While it recognises the need for follow-up and perhaps future intervention in some cases, it also addresses the issue of effective use of resources, for example through packages of care.
- It is suited to different types of disability. Individuals are homogeneous in their EDS aversion.
- Although teamwork is touted in the literature there is little evidence to suggest that it is a functioning viable tool. However, the often arbitrary boundaries in EDS necessitate that we work co-operatively together to provide solutions to these problems. Working in teams is always a challenge, and programmes such as Fun with Food provide a basis for clinicians to move forward together to address the needs of individuals with EDS difficulties.
- Previous feeding studies targeting one area of intervention, for example oral motor dysfunction, are not encouraging. Oral motor management is the most common therapeutic intervention for children with EDS difficulties and efficacy studies have been limited predominantly to non-randomised studies. Some examples follow.

It may be that intervention has been less successful in many cases, as some authors (Gisel 1994) have suggested, because it adapted a singular approach to a multifactorial clinical problem. A holistic approach based on a global view of the child's problems (via an interdisciplinary approach which recognises that EDS problems can be influenced by medical, physical, cognitive, sensory, interaction *and* behavioural issues) may be more effective.

Table 6: Oral motor interventions in EDS

Finding	Authors
Oral motor interventions can improve oral motor function, but have not been shown to be effective in promoting feeding efficiency or weight gain.	Gisel et al (1996) Rogers (2004)
Study with control and treatment periods. Significant improvement in the following eating parameters: spoon-feeding; chewing; swallowing. Treatment may help children ingest food more competently (ie less spillage) but not increase weight.	Gisel et al (1996)
Demonstrated no change in oral motor function or weight gain during 9 weeks of sensorimotor treatment in children with developmental disabilities.	Ottenbacher et al (1981, 1983)
Limited gains in oral motor skills following 20 weeks of non-randomised sensorimotor treatment. 'Oral motor therapy may have to be combined with oral caloric supplementation.'	Gisel (1994)
10–20 weeks of oral sensorimotor therapy did not impact on eating efficiency in children with cerebral palsy. Children also showed no catch-up in growth. Findings suggest that eating efficiency is not a good estimate of treatment outcome but rather a diagnostic indicator of the severity of eating impairment.	Gisel et al (1995)

Multiple targets in EDS therapy

Recent research suggests that multiple targets in EDS therapy may prove more effective (see Table 7).

So aversion should not simply be interpreted as a behavioural problem; the origin of the behaviour may be more complex. In such cases a multicomponent programme may best meet the needs of these children. The focus in Fun with Food on carer training (discussed in Chapter 3), and interaction therapy in particular, reflects more recent developments in clinical intervention (eg Mathews et al, 1997), although there is the need for more clinical evidence.

The intensive nature of the treatment may also be relevant. Byars et al (2003) found that multiple daily treatments provide a consistent setting for diminishing severe mealtime behavioural resistance.

Table 7: Multicomponent interventions in EDS

Area	Finding	Authors
Swallow function	Non-randomised therapy trial over 18 months. Cerebral palsied subjects. Results suggest that the 'profoundly retarded cerebral palsied patient is capable of making gains in swallow function'. Treatment included dietary modifications, oral motor treatment and thermal stimulation.	Helfrish-Miller et al (1986)
Pulmonary function/ Weight gain	Examined whether pulmonary function would improve following one year of intervention with optimal positioning, control of gastro-oesophageal reflux and use of food textures that would minimise aspiration from swallowing. All children gained sufficient weight to maintain growth trajectories but only one (who went from oral to tube feed) showed gain in length. Control of aspiration permitted a clinically significant improvement in their pulmonary function.	Gisel et al (2003)

Recently, single case studies (Guttentag & Hammer, 2000; Farrell et al, 2001; Randall et al, 2002) have shown successful outcomes in developing oral eating in tube feeders, and there has also been some randomised controlled trial (Benoit et al, 2000) and non-randomised (Byars et al, 2003) evidence.

The benefits of a multicomponent programme

In Fun with Food, use of a number of functional measures to evaluate progress and initial research outcomes (McCurtin, Kennedy & Walsh, unpublished) shows significant changes in food approach behaviour, oral-nutritional behaviour, the number and frequency of foods and drinks tolerated and the number of flavours tried. Of the four (of nine) clients who were totally dependent on tube feeding at the study commencement, three came off tubes, with the other one minimally supported by tube. There was therefore:

- Reduction in tube-feed dependence
- Maintenance of body weight
- Long-term gains (assessed at 12 months)
- Increased comfort levels for aversive eaters at the table

- Improvement in oral-nutritional behaviours (location of food contact)
- Increase in the range of foods taken.

The initial indications are that multicomponent-focused interventions such as the Fun with Food programme can be successful and implemented on an outpatient basis. It may be that either the intensive nature of these programmes or the support given to carers may be the essential criteria for success, rather than the specific nature or content of the programme itself. Treatment in this manner can also be cost efficient. Based on staff and tube-feed formula costs in 2004, the outlay for one course for five children can be recouped by the successful transition of only one child from tube to oral feeds.

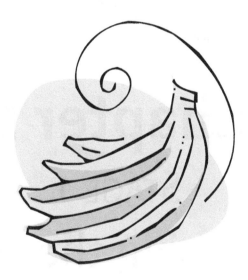

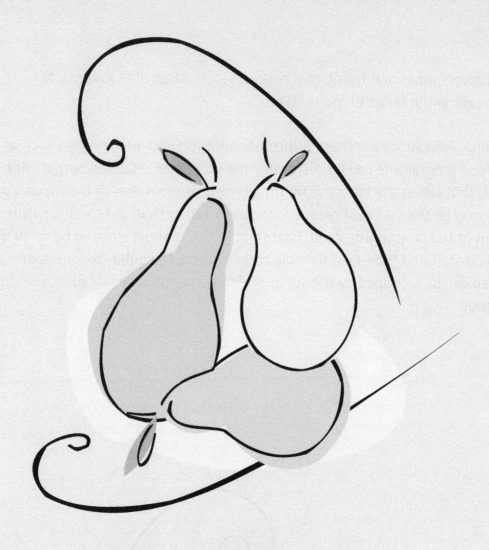

Chapter 2

STAGE 1

Assessing the child

Assessments can be conducted by different professionals and may reflect the role of the profession in particular or the interests of the specific clinician. For example, oral motor skills are always assessed by the speech & language therapists, and the child's nutritional status by the dietitian. Assessments are typically carried out in two stages: pre-contact forms which are sent to carers for filling in (eg Case History Form), and Assessment Day, where children attend multiple appointments for assessment of individual areas (eg sensory skills).

The aims of assessment for the programme are to:

1 Select appropriate candidates for Fun with Food intervention, ie to determine the presence or absence of an eating & drinking & swallowing (EDS) aversion.
2 Determine the child's suitability for both Fun before Food (pre-feeding skills) and Eating, Drinking and Swallowing elements of the course by evaluating support skills, such as oral motor function and sensory processing abilities, in addition to EDS skills.
3 Ensure the child's medical status is stable and any appropriate medical management is carried out (eg medication for reflux).
4 Assess the child's nutritional status and ensure their nutritional stability.
5 Group possible candidates to best group fit.
6 Confirm carer commitment to all aspects of the programme.

Pre-assessment contact

Prior to assessment of the child, information should be obtained from the carer by the clinician. This helps to provide a baseline for intervention and ensures that essential medical investigations and management are not neglected. Five forms (listed below) and a covering letter (to be found at the end of this chapter) are sent to the carers, who are required to complete them:

1 Case History Form (Form 2.1)
2 Food Diary (Forms 2.2, 2.3)
3 Carer construction of Eating & Drinking & Swallowing Problem (Form 2.5)
4 Sensory Profile Carer Questionnaire (Form 2.18)
5 Videotaping Permission Form (Form 2.4).

Table 8: Pre-assessment forms

Form	Notes
Case History Form	This form is comprehensive in its inclusion of nutritional, medical, oral motor, communication, independence and sensory areas. It will provide team members with a complete overview of child-specific EDS issues.
Food Diary	The sample Food Diary and blank Food Diary should be sent together, to provide the carer with guidelines for filling out the child's Food Diary. The carer should fill out three days' worth of diary, two weekdays and one week-end day, to provide the clinician with as accurate a representation as possible. It aims to provide nutritional, environmental and equipment information.
Carer construction of EDS problem	Provides carer with an opportunity to clearly identify concerns. Facilitates holistic approach to treatment.
The Sensory Profile: Caregiver Questionnaire (Dunn, 1999a)	Judgement-based questionnaire used to elicit sensory processing skills and deficits.
Videotaping Permission Form	Obtains consent for videotaping of sessions.

Essential form-filling

The Case History Form and the Food Diary are the two forms which are **mandatory**. Should the carer require help to complete these forms, extra time needs to be allotted for this purpose, either on the Assessment Day or through a home visit.

Experience has shown that videotaping a 'typical' home mealtime does not significantly enhance the clinician's understanding of the child, nor does it elicit any information or insight that cannot be obtained elsewhere during the programme. Videotaping is therefore confined to the clinic.

It is important not to overload the carer with paperwork before intervention has commenced. The clinician should therefore use their knowledge of the family in deciding which forms to send out for completion prior to the Assessment Day. Other forms such as the Independence Questionnaire and Tastes & Textures Questionnaire can be also sent at this time. Alternatively, they can be completed by carers with a clinician on the Assessment Day.

Copies of the forms can be found at the end of the chapter (see page 45).

Assessments

Team members (speech & language therapist, dietitian, occupational therapist etc) can elect to assess the children within their own individual clinic time. The team can then meet to discuss results and decide on the suitability of individual children for the programme. However, given the number of appointments necessary to obtain a comprehensive overview of the child's EDS problems, a day of assessments may be more feasible for the family and team.

A sample timetable of a typical Assessment Day is shown in Appendix 1 (Form A1.2). This illustrates how a co-ordinator can organise the various team members and children to make the most effective use of time.

Suggested assessment areas are:

- Interaction (Video assessment)
- Nutrition
- Taste & Textures
- Oral motor skills
- Sensory processing
- Independence
- Medical.

Video assessments

Analysis of the videotaped evidence includes:

1 Carer–child interaction during an eating activity
2 Food approach behaviours
3 Recording of basic EDS skills.

The author makes no apologies for the focus on interaction skills and the behaviourist approach to intervention. This approach reflects difficulties that children with disabilities experience around the control of eating and drinking (fewer choices offered, limited communication skills, frustration etc), and also those of their carers (eg anxiety about nutrition, overcompensation etc), which may serve to compound the EDS problem. Luiselli (1989) reports that many feeding problems develop initially, and/or are maintained subsequently, by the interaction between organic and non-organic factors. Given that normal mealtimes provide numerous social and communication opportunities, focus on the interaction at mealtimes is pivotal to successful development of EDS skills and the enhancement of the child–carer relationship.

The videotaped session should show the child eating (with carer present) and should last no more than 15 minutes. Although this session can never be typical because it is conducted in a clinic room, the information it provides is sufficient to determine the presence and extent of EDS aversion and child–carer interaction styles. A sample Carer–Child Interaction Summary Form (2.12) can be found at the end of the chapter. The purpose of this session is to:

- Determine the presence of EDS aversion
- Define the degree of EDS aversion (total or selective)
- Obtain a baseline of child behaviour and food approach behaviour
- Obtain a baseline of carer style of interaction and management, and child's response to same
- Obtain an overview of EDS skills.

The clinician should have a range of food and drink available to facilitate this session (an assortment of which is identified in Chapter 5), particularly in case the carer forgets, or has not understood, the instructions. However, because of the nature of aversion (selectivity in eating), and to provide a more accurate impression of the child's EDS skills and food approach behaviour, the carer is asked to bring to the session a typical representation of the child's food including:

- Preferred foods, at least one solid and one drink. Preferred foods are defined as those a child will either request voluntarily or accept without being coerced or behaving negatively as a result.
- Non-preferred foods, at least one solid and one drink. Non-preferred foods typically result in refusal or negative behaviours.

In making the video, the carer should be informed of the following points.

- Be as natural as possible. The video needs to be as accurate a representation of as 'normal' a situation as possible. Do not encourage the child to be on their best behaviour because of the video – the clinicians need to see what really happens. Treat the child's behaviour as if they were at home. Use the same language, same reactions and so on.
- Do not use statements such as 'Eat for the lady', 'The lady wants to see if you will eat for mummy'.
- Do not forewarn the child about videotaping.

■ Give the child preferred and non-preferred food and drink items. Preferred items are those which they will take relatively willingly – if they have none, this is acceptable. Non-preferred foods are those which the child typically refuses when offered. It is informative for the clinicians to see how the child copes in these different situations. Offer one food (solid) item and one drink for both the preferred and non-preferred categories.

■ The video should last 15 minutes. The carer and child can leave before then if the child has finished eating and drinking, as the child is not required to eat a specific amount.

The forms (2.6–2.11) which can be used for these video assessments and completed by the clinician are identified in Table 9 below and guidelines on how to use them are provided. Not all forms are essential. The clinician can decide which are necessary based on the individual child's presentation and needs. Form blanks follow at the end of the chapter (pages 65–70).

Table 9: Areas of video assessment

Description	Guidelines for recording behaviours
Food approach behaviour (Form 2.6) Behaviours which precede actual oral contact with food. The two main areas identified here are: 1. *Sitting with ease*: Defined as in the chair, whole body facing table and food, without significant gap between chair and table. Not protesting for more than 10 seconds verbally or non-verbally. 2. *Intentional eating*: Includes taking spoon from plate/lifting cup to swallow, ie actual eating behaviour, not 'messing' with food, eg stirring repetitively, which can be defined as a non-intentional eating behaviour.	Behaviours are recorded based on time. The total time is recorded, divided into time for preferred and non-preferred items, and entered into the appropriate frequency box. Tick the appropriate column for each section after watching the video. The clinician may want to review the videotape a second time.

continued →

Table 9: *continued*

Description	Guidelines for recording behaviours
Oral-nutritional behaviour (Form 2.7) Based on the food's actual destination – the oral cavity. They are recorded by the location/contact of the body part with food and the action involved therein. This section is designed to recognise the progression many individuals with extreme oral aversion must make prior to achieving oral eating. Not to do so would be to understate and undervalue the effort made by these individuals and undermine the role other factors have in the area of eating and drinking aversion. See Table 10 for definitions of oral-nutritional behaviour.	Recorded based on frequency of occurrence for preferred and non-preferred items. Tick the appropriate column for each section after watching the 15 minute video. You may want to review the videotape a second time. A guide to use of the frequency ratings is as follows. It is generally found that once children progress to 9 and 10 contacts, the behaviour then becomes normalised and frequency counts are not necessary. *Never* = behaviour did not occur during videotape *Sometimes* = behaviour observed 1–2 times *Occasionally* = behaviour observed 3–5 times *Frequently* = behaviour observed 5–9 times *Constantly* = behaviour observed 10+ times.
Flavours & Consistencies Record (Form 2.8) This area attempts only to summarise the range (flavours/tastes and consistencies/textures) of oral intake and to chart progress of same throughout the programme. Progress should be defined by increase in the breadth of the range of foods taken. Definitions are provided in Table 11.	Recorded based on frequency of occurrence for preferred and non-preferred items. Tick the appropriate column for each section after watching the video. A food item finished should receive automatically a '*constantly*' grading. Use the same frequency ratings as for the previous section.

continued ➜

Table 9: *continued*

Description	Guidelines for recording behaviours
EDS Script (Form 2.9) Used to keep a record of the language used in the EDS activity. It can be useful particularly to get an idea of the dominance in verbal communication – who talks most – and the degree of food-related verbalisations during eating. This form can be used in a carer activity during the care element of the programme (see Chapter 3). The form also has value in charting interaction styles such as questions (many carers tend to ask their children's 'permission' when they offer food – thereby offering the opportunity to refuse).	The language used by both carer and child is recorded verbatim. Speaker refers to the child or carer or other person. Statement is the accurate written evidence of what exactly was said. Note refers to additional information which helps interpret the verbal information, eg non-verbal cues. Statements should be scripted in sequence as they occur.
EDS Script Summary Count (Form 2.10) Adds simple interpretation to EDS script. Can be subjective in nature, such as 'negative' comments. Any interpretation of the information obtained should be made with this in mind. Clinicians should add-in relevant categories based on individual child–carer interaction sequences.	Words in total and words per minutes are counted and tabulated. Child and carer statements are allocated to various categories such as repetitions, questions, utterances related to food, use of praise/reinforcement, negotiations and negative statements.
Child–Carer Interaction Summary (Form 2.11) Analysis of 'constructive' and 'non-constructive' behaviours. Constructive behaviours are those which should contribute to successful eating and drinking for the child, eg smiling, use of praise. Non-constructive behaviours are the opposite; they have a potentially negative impact, and may include behaviours such as shouting at the child. The clinician should review the videotape and fill in the form to summarise interaction styles and behaviours observed during the EDS video. This can be used both to measure change and to facilitate carer development. See Table 2.4 for examples of behaviours.	Record child and carer behaviours which are both constructive and non-constructive to the development of the child's EDS skills. Behaviours can be both verbal and non-verbal.

Table 10: Definitions of oral-nutritional behaviour

Location of food contact	Behaviour	Outcome
Non-oral contact	Touched food or drink with hands or utensil	Non-nutritional
Pre-oral	Touched/tasted food or drink with lips or tongue	Non-nutritional
Intraoral	Took food or drink into mouth	Lips closed or food visible in mouth Nutritional or non-nutritional
Pharyngeal	Swallowed food or drink	Mouth empty Nutritional

Table 11 provides a sample of definitions. Clinicians may refer to their own professional guidelines to provide internal consistency.

Table 11: Food range definitions

Food	Definition	Examples
	Flavours/Tastes	
Bland food	Food with no defined taste, ie unsalted, unsweetened	Porridge, milk
Savoury food	Food with tartness – non-spicy, non-sweet	Dinners, pasta, soups, vegetables
Sweet food	Food with added or natural sugars	Sugared cereals, banana
Spicy food	Added spices	Curry
Bitter food	Unpleasant/harsh to the taste	Lemon
	Consistencies/Textures	
Liquid	Un-thickened liquids, move freely and quickly	Water, sodas
Purée	Food that moves quickly to slowly – not solid, not liquid	Yoghurt, 4-month baby jars
Mashed texture	Food that is mashed	Potato mash, turnip mash
Roughly mashed	Food that is mashed with small soft lumps	As above
Mixed texture	Food with more than one texture, eg lumps and purées	Beans, stews
Soft separate lumps	Solid separate foods which should be chewed	Banana pieces, cooked/ semi-cooked carrots
Hard separate lumps	Hard separate foods which require diagonal/ rotary chewing	Biscuits, raw vegetables

Nutritional assessment

Marie Kennedy

In working with children with disabilities, the nutritional component of both the assessment and intervention programmes must be emphasised due to the significance of nutritional issues for this population (Sullivan et al, 2000). This holds true for aversion as well. The dietetic part of the assessment evaluates current nutritional intake (eg energy, protein, iron, calcium and vitamin C), weight, height, oral vs tube intake and so on (Krick et al, 1991). The purpose of the nutritional assessment is to ensure nutritional stability, provide a baseline for monitoring weight during the programme and ensure balanced nutrition.

What the assessment should cover
Nutritional assessment should be undertaken by a qualified dietitian/nutritionist and include details on:

- Weight
- Height
- Ideal body weight, calculated as a percentage of body weight in relation to the child's height (Krick et al, 1996)
- Dietary deficiencies. The Food Diary can be utilised to assess if any dietary deficiencies are present as this will provide a good basis for the evaluation. The dietitian will adjust the child's diet accordingly, for example check tolerance of sip-feed supplements and check the necessity for supplements
- Tube feeds. A record of the tube-feeding regime will be taken and ways of reducing or removing the tube-feed will be evaluated in the context of the programme and the child's needs. Possible alternatives to tube feeds should be discussed with the carers and supplements may be trialled. This facilitates the clinician in setting goals for the programme that are practical, and that can be realistically carried out by both the carers and child. On tube-feed reductions the dietitian will match calories, protein, vitamins and minerals with their equivalent in oral food or oral nutritional supplements, and will always meet nutritional requirements according to appropriate professionally agreed guidelines.

To facilitate monitoring, the dietitian can utilise a rating scale such as the Nutritional Intake Form outlined at the end of the chapter (Form 2.13).

Tastes & Textures Questionnaire

Trish Morrison

The Tastes & Textures Questionnaire (Form 2.14 on pages 73–77; Tables 12, 13) is designed to determine:

- Foods and drinks the child can tolerate
- Consistencies of tolerated foods and drinks
- Tastes the child has experienced, and
- Food or drink consistencies that the carer/child would avoid and why.

Koontz Lowman and McKeever Murphy (1999) state that children will often refuse food because of the effects of touch, taste, temperature and texture – they may be responding to any one of these sensations. Using the questionnaire helps to:

1 Identify the number of foods and drinks the child will tolerate, albeit in very small quantities, the criterion being that the child swallows one-quarter of a teaspoon of the food or fluid.
2 Consider how frequently the foods and drinks are taken.
3 Examine the tastes the child has experienced (salty, bitter, sour, sweet and spicy) – a lick being the basic expectation here.

The food identified via the questionnaire would not contribute to nutritional intake given the small quantities, but the information is useful in obtaining descriptive information about food consumption patterns and may be used in conjunction with food records to provide a more complete picture of usual intake. The information obtained appears sensitive to charting small changes in food and drink intake and taste experience.

Additional questions serve to augment the sensory information available and provide information required for the carer experiential exercise in the Food for Thought carer programme (see Chapter 3). Also included in the questionnaire is a general question regarding negative reactions to food/drink-related experiences other than eating, for example the sound of food and drink being prepared. This information is sought to broaden the understanding of the child's aversion, and to see how it correlates with information from the Sensory Assessment.

Table 12: Notes on the Tastes & Textures Questionnaire

About consistencies/textures

- Textures are considered important, as having chewable foods in your diet 'helps to provide a base for muscle growth in the oral/facial structures' (Koontz Lowman & McKeever Murphy, 1999), varied textures being necessary to provide the oral stimulation required by the sensory system.

- Identifying the food textures tolerated helps to inform therapy goals. Different textures can be introduced gradually in conjunction with an oral motor programme which will promote the skills needed to cope with the food textures.

- The consistency of each food or drink tolerated is recorded. Broadly speaking the consistencies follow a developmental sequence: Liquids, Purée (no lumps), Mash (no lumps), Roughly mashed (small lumps in with the mash), Soft separate lumps (eg cooked carrots, banana, pear or sausage), and hard lumps (eg apple or raw carrot).

About tastes/flavours

- Information is sought regarding the tastes the child has experienced: sweet, salty, sour, bitter and spicy.

- Spicy is included because children who are hyposensitive to taste often prefer spicy food or stronger tastes (Koontz Lowman & McKeever Murphy, 1999).

- Taste is experienced on the tongue: hence, for example, a lick of salty food is accepted as the salty taste having been experienced. There are many other factors that influence our experience of taste. Dunn Klein and Evans Morris (1999) mention our age, intactness of the taste buds and the olfactory system as well as an emotional component (ie our past experience), but these are not addressed here for the purposes of this programme.

Table 13: Tastes & Textures Questionnaire recording guidelines

Question	Recording guideline	Scoring
Q1 & Q2	Note in the space provided each food or drink tolerated. Record how frequently the food is consumed (monthly, weekly, 2 times a week, 3–5 times a week or daily). Also record the consistency of the food, referring to the instructions that accompany the questionnaire. For detailed information on how to record the consistency see the instruction sheet that accompanies the questionnaire.	Each food or drink item tolerated receives a score of 1.0. The frequency scores are numbered 1–5 (where 1 = monthly and 5 = daily). These frequency scores are summated. Thus a child that eats two foods (score 2.0), one of them daily (0.5) and the other weekly (0.2), would receive a score of 2.7.
Q3 & Q4	Mark a tick in the box for all consistencies that a carer would avoid giving the child. Record their reasons for avoiding that consistency.	The total possible score is 5 for question 3, and 3 for question 4. 1 point is allocated for each consistency that would be avoided; thus if a carer would only present purée (no lumps) the score for question 3 would be 4.
Q5	Mark a tick in the box for each taste that the child has experienced, giving an example of the food.	There is a total possible score of 5 with 1 point being allocated for each taste the child has experienced (a lick).
Q6	Mark a tick in the box for each item that applies to the client, then describe the reaction in the space provided.	The information is noted because it addresses some broader sensory issues, but it is not scored.
Q7 & Q8	Only complete these questions if the plan is to include a carer experiential exercise to simulate aversion in the carer element of the programme.	The information is noted but not scored.

Oral Motor Skills assessment

Petro Van Deventer

This section evaluates oral and facial sensation, tone and function, and eating functions including swallow, chewing and biting. This determines the presence and impact of any oral motor dysfunction on EDS, and facilitates targeting the individual's programme in both the pre-feeding Fun before Food and Eating & Drinking & Swallowing programme sections. It also helps when advising carers on suitable consistencies. Children with oral motor dysfunction require mandatory attendance at the pre-feeding programme in order to facilitate their approach to eating and drinking.

Oral motor skills follow a successive pattern of development (Frick et al, 1996) to achieve the strength, mobility and co-ordination of movement required for efficient eating, drinking and swallowing. A child needs to develop both motor- and sensory-based skills; limitations in either of these areas can contribute to aversive feeding behaviour (Overland, 2001).

Oral motor skills are assessed by observing the structure and movement patterns of the jaw, cheeks, lips, tongue, palate and teeth. The child should be observed at rest and during the performance of oral imitation and oral motor tasks. This will provide valuable information regarding muscle strength, co-ordination, dissociation and range of movement in the jaw, lips, cheeks and tongue.

Isolated movements related to feeding, such as tongue-tip elevation or tongue lateralisation, can also be assessed during the performance of oral imitation tasks. As 'sensation stimulates movement', which in turn 'facilitates and shapes oral stabilisation and differentiation skills' (Jared et al, 2000), the acceptance of touch would be an important factor to consider during assessment and treatment of oral motor concerns. So, prior to implementation of a treatment programme, the child's response to touch should be determined to ensure appropriate sensory input, as treatment strategies for a child with hypersensitivity would differ from that of a child with hyposensitivity (Macky, 1996).

Children who have had limited oral experiences may present with unrefined oral motor patterns during eating and drinking. They may react with aversive behaviour towards EDS if they do not have the necessary skills to support oral feeding. Also, opportunities to observe oral movement patterns may be restricted as the children may not be feeding orally. The carer can supply valuable information both about a child's previous oral experiences and the difficulties a child may have relating to oral EDS. In addition to carer information, observation of a child's oral motor skills during a meal is essential, and the videotape of the EDS assessment session can be used to this end. This will ensure that the goals devised will facilitate the 'practicing of oral motor patterns that is both appropriate within the child's oral motor development and would also allow advancement to the next oral motor milestone/skill' (Kerwin et al, 1992). The clinician can also engage the child in a series of oral activities where a reasonable amount of information can be obtained. By observing a 'variety of responses that the child is exhibiting', the clinician can 'decide which responses are important to inhibit and which responses are important to facilitate' (Chapman Bahr, 2001).

Guidelines for assessment

1   Sensation
    ■ Introduce a hand puppet to the child. Let the puppet touch the child's hand, shoulder, face and lips. Note sensitivity. If the child rejects touch on the face, omit the next step. If touch is accepted, move to the next step.
    ■ If the child tolerates touch with the puppet, put on surgical gloves, and with the hands, uses gentle firm presses to massage the child's face. Start at the tempero-mandibular joint and gradually move towards the mouth, around the mouth and then, on the lips, use index, middle and ring finger to apply firm presses around and on the lips. Document responses.
    ■ Follow the sequence outlined in the Oral Motor Exam Form 2 (page 81). Use a rolling motion when using a tool. When stimulating the tongue, begin at the front and move backwards gradually. Do the same with the palate. Start with the alveolar ridge and move backwards. Document the child's response.

2   Observation of oral structures at rest
    ■ Follow the checklist in Oral Motor Exam Forms 1 or 2 (pages 78–86) and document the appearance of oral structures at rest. More information, for example the status of the back molars, length of the frenulum and so on, may be documented when evaluating the position and movement of oral structures during EDS and oral activities.

3   Position and movement patterns (non-nutritive)
    The child is requested to engage in a series of oral imitation and oral motor tasks to evaluate the position and movement patterns of oral structures during tasks that do not require the manipulation of a bolus. These activities are introduced first to determine the child's strength and co-ordination of oral movements.
    ■ To document the movement patterns present in the lips, the child is requested to imitate and hold a kissing posture with the lips, then maintain a smiling posture.

The child is then asked to puff their cheeks and their ability to maintain adequate lip seal is documented. To investigate lip rounding, the child is requested to blow bubbles. The final task is to hold a spatula horizontally between the lips (without biting onto it). Document the length of time the child is able to maintain this posture. It is important to make sure that the child is able to breathe through their nose when introducing this task, which will provide information regarding lip closure as well as jaw stability and jaw–lip dissociation (Rosenfeld-Johnson, 2001).

- The movement patterns in the jaw are recorded during the following oral motor and imitation tasks. The child is requested to open and close his mouth slowly. The grading of jaw movements is documented. The child is requested to clatter his teeth, mimicking coldness. The co-ordination of repetitive movement is documented. A Chewy Tube® is introduced to the child. A puppet can be used to introduce the tool and to demonstrate the activity. If the child accepts the tool, the child is requested to place the tube between his back molars on the one side and is then asked to bite down. The status of his natural bite is documented. Next the child is asked to chew on the tube on each side and the number of repetitions and the preferred side for chewing are documented.

- The movement patterns observed in the tongue are documented during the imitation of specific tasks. The child is requested to stick his tongue out, to elevate and depress the tongue and also to move it from side to side. Weaknesses or limited range of movements are noted. Associated movements such as movement of the jaw, head or other body parts during these tasks should also be documented.

4 Position and movement patterns (nutritive)

Use the video recording of the carer–child EDS activity to fill out this part of the assessment. The aim is to determine the child's current developmental level of eating in order to devise appropriate goals to refine current skills and to develop skills appropriately. The effectiveness of a child's oral motor skills plays an important role in the child's ability to eat and drink safely. After completing the assessment, use information obtained to determine whether oral motor skills observed would support safe feeding. Describe specific skills that need to be developed to improve safe and efficient eating, drinking and swallowing.

- Document the utensils used for eating.

- Note and document the mobility, co-ordination and strength of oral structures during biting and chewing. Observe whether movements are graded and symmetrical. If there is loss of food during feeding, note whether the individual is aware of it and the reason for same (eg lip seal, poor bolus movement intraorally).

■ During chewing, note if there is a preferred side for chewing and the developmental level of jaw movement (munching/diagonal/rotary movement etc). Also note the size of bites. Tick appropriate boxes while observing the intraoral movements during biting and chewing and swallowing.

■ During eating, drinking and swallowing, note the co-ordination between oral, pharyngeal and respiratory components.

■ Document the efficiency of protective reflexes. Examine non-nutritive and nutritive cough and swallow functions.

Two Oral Motor Exam (OME) options forms (Forms 2.15 and 2.16) and a Summary Sheet (Form 2.17) follow at the end of the chapter.

Sensory Processing assessment

Jeni Malone

In addressing the problems of children with aversive EDS problems, the approach adopted needs to incorporate sensory processing skills. Sensory input is important to normal development (Ayres, 1979). A child's ability to process sensory information can greatly impact functional abilities in daily tasks including EDS (Bundy, 1991; Dunn, 1997) and children with sensory processing difficulties may be more sensitive to EDS problems because of the high concentration of receptors in the oral and facial areas. Children with sensory processing issues require mandatory attendance at the pre-feeding programme in order to facilitate their approach to eating and drinking.

The aims of this section are to:

1 Measure the child's overall sensory processing abilities.
2 Identify levels of participation in tactile/sensory play and identify specific reactions to different tactile stimuli (especially in relation to the hands and face).
3 Develop a therapy programme that will address some of the specific difficulties highlighted in point 2.
4 Identify any changes in 1 and/or 2 after the programme, and identify any link to changes in EDS behaviour.

Sensory integration theory identifies five distinct sensory systems – proprioceptive, vestibular, tactile, visual and auditory. It also states that these systems interact to produce behavioural outcomes, for example the vestibular system is thought to have a role in modulation of all other sensory systems (Ayres, 1979).

Sensory defensiveness is often found in more than one sensory system (Kinnealy et al, 1995; Wilbarger, 1995). The term sensory defensiveness is used to describe a:

> constellation of symptoms that are related to aversive or defensive reactions to non-noxious stimuli across one or more sensory systems. It is an over reaction of our normal protective senses. Individuals with sensory defensiveness have their own response style. There may be patterns of avoidance, sensory seeking, fear, anxiety or even aggression. These symptoms fluctuate widely and can be misidentified as only emotionally based. *(Wilbarger & Wilbarger, 2001)*

Some children with EDS problems display behaviours suggestive of defensiveness and/or other modulation difficulties. Different types of modulation disorders have been identified, with behavioural outcomes varying depending on which sensory system (or systems) is affected (Bundy & Murray, 1991). Sensory modulation disorder can manifest in the child's over- or under-responsiveness to, or displaying a fluctuating response to, sensory input (Dunn, 1997; Wilbarger & Wilbarger, 2001). Four identified types of modulation disorder are:

- Sensory defensiveness. This includes tactile defensiveness but has been described in other sensory systems
- Gravitational insecurity
- Aversive responses to movement
- Under-responsiveness (Bundy & Murray, 1991).

Assessment consists of:

1 History taking
   - The Sensory Profile: Caregiver Questionnaire (Dunn, 1999a) can be forwarded to carers and the completed form brought to the Assessment Day. Any queries or difficulties with any of the items can be addressed at the assessment stage. The Sensory Profile is a judgement-based questionnaire used to measure a child's sensory processing abilities. It provides information on the child's sensory preferences and level of responsiveness to sensory input in general, through observation and recording of specific reactions to a range of tactile/sensory activities. It can be used to indicate the level of functional performance in different activities and to indicate meaningful clusters of behaviour suggesting difficulties in processing specific types of sensory information.

This questionnaire is not suitable for test-retest and mapping progress. It can be re-administered after a period of time if the clinician wants a more recent view of daily behaviour and functional abilities at home. This can be useful in some cases in this programme but in others, as it is a subjective questionnaire, results can reflect a change in caregiver rather than child, for example due to carers' increased level of understanding about behaviours that were previously unrecognised.

■ Evaluate the case history for risk factors such as an insult to the developing neurological system at birth, in utero or when the system is vulnerable; any sensory deprivation(eg extended long-stay in hospital), any noxious sensory events such as repeated medical procedures (eg nasogastric tube routing, reflux).

2 Observation & probes
Many occupational therapy departments have their own criterion-referenced checklists/assessments for looking at a child's sensory processing skills. The one used here is one such example (Form 2.18, see page 45). Clinicians should feel free to take ideas from this or create one suited to their situation, resources and individual needs. The purpose of this checklist is to provide a framework for the presentation of a variety of sensory input to the child in a structured manner. All sessions are videotaped to enable the clinician to review the child's behaviour in more detail later, present the same input in the same manner at a later date, and map changes for the clinician and carer, allowing for factors such as the child's maturity and level of ease in surroundings.

The sections of this checklist relating to oral sensation should be completed by the speech & language therapist and results of the sensory assessment must be clearly communicated to other team members to ensure expectations placed on the child are appropriate and achievable. This is especially important for some of the normalisation activities.

Guidelines on presentation and scoring of materials for sensory activities
Guidelines for presentation and scoring of some of the activities are given in Table 14. All activities should be scored in a similar manner.

Please note that this is not a full sensory integration assessment and, if one is warranted, a child should be seen by a fully qualified sensory integration therapist. If a child is already seeing such a therapist or has a full programme drawn up, changes/additions should not be made without full liaison with the primary therapist.

Table 14: Guidelines for sensory assessment

Activity	Recording
Vestibular Linear – up/down: Bouncing on ball, sitting, clinician supporting at hips. Say 'We are going to bounce on the ball'.	1 – Child does not complete activity 2 – Child assumes seated position on ball (with assistance) 3 – Child completes 5 assisted bounces on third attempt/presentation 4 – Child completes 5 assisted bounces on second attempt/presentation 5 – Child completes 5 assisted bounces on first attempt/presentation.
Orientation – prone/upright: Prone on ball, rolling forwards to ground, reach for object (skittle) and back. Say 'We are going to lie on the ball and knock the skittles'.	1 – Child does not complete activity 2 – Child assumes prone position on ball (with assistance) 3 – Child completes roll forward, reach object & back on third attempt 4 – Child completes roll forward, reach object & back on second attempt 5 – Child completes roll forward, reach object & back on first attempt.
Rotary – spin: Sitting on office chair and clinician spinning it. Say 'We are going to spin around on the chair'.	1 – Child does not complete activity 2 – Child assumes seated position on chair (with assistance) 3 – Child completes one full spin on third attempt 4 – Child completes one full spin on second attempt 5 – Child completes one full spin on first attempt.
Tactile Processing Haptic/Facial: Gritty – sand → hands: Child shown toys buried in sand. Say 'We are going to find the toys in the sand'.	1 – Child does not complete activity 2 – Therapist rakes child's hand through sand 3 – Therapist places own hand in sand and child then completes 4 – Child places hand in sand with auditory cue 5 – Child places hand in sand upon presentation.

continued →

Table 14: *continued*

Activity	Recording
Sticky – putty → hands: Child presented with gloop/putty. Say 'We are going to play with the putty'.	1 – Child does not complete activity 2 – Clinician places putty in child's hand (3 attempts) 3 – Clinician picks up putty and child then picks it up 4 – Child picks putty up with auditory cue or touches upon presentation 5 – Child picks putty up upon presentation.
Soft/fluffy → hands: Child presented with soft/fluffy puppets. Say 'We are going to play with the puppets'.	1 – Child does not complete activity 2 – Clinician touches puppet to child's hand (3 attempts) 3 – Clinician handles puppet, and child then handles puppet 4 – Child handles puppet with auditory cue 5 – Child handles puppet upon presentation.
Soft/fluffy → face: Say 'The puppet wants to kiss you on the cheek'.	1 – Child does not complete activity 2 – Clinician touches puppet to child's cheek (3 attempts) 3 – Clinician handles puppet to own cheek and child then completes 4 – Child touches puppet to cheek with auditory cue 5 – Child touches puppet to cheek upon presentation.
Vibration → hands: Child shown vibrating 'gator' toy (vibrating toy). Say 'Look, gator is cold'.	1 – Child does not complete activity 2 – Clinician touches 'gator' to child's hand (3 attempts) 3 – Clinician touches 'gator', and child then touches 4 – Child touches 'gator' with auditory cue 5 – Child touches 'gator' upon presentation.
Vibration → face: Say 'Gator wants to kiss you on the cheek'.	1 – Child does not complete activity 2 – Clinician touches 'gator' to child's cheek (3 attempts) 3 – Clinician touches 'gator' to own cheek and child then completes 4 – Child touches 'gator' to cheek with auditory cue 5 – Child touches 'gator' to cheek upon presentation.

continued →

Table 14: *continued*

Activity	Recording
Vibration → lips: Say 'Gator wants to kiss you on the lips'.	1 – Child does not complete activity 2 – Clinician touches 'gator' to child's lips (3 attempts) 3 – Clinician touches 'gator' to own lips and child then completes 4 – Child touches 'gator' to lips with auditory cue 5 – Child touches 'gator' to lips upon presentation.
Wet/liquid – paint → hands: Child given paints in container with paper and no brushes. Say 'We are going to paint with our hand'.	1 – Child does not complete activity 2 – Clinician touches child's hand to paint (3 attempts) 3 – Clinician touches paint and child then touches paint 4 – Child touches paint with auditory cue 5 – Child touches paint upon presentation.
Wet/liquid – water → hands/arms: Child given basin of soapy water. Say 'We are going to wash our hands'.	1 – Child does not complete activity 2 – Clinician puts child's hand in water (3 attempts) 3 – Clinician puts hand in water and child then completes 4 – Child puts hand in water with auditory cue 5 – Child puts hand in water upon presentation.
Wet/liquid – water → face: Say 'We are going to wash our face'.	1 – Child does not complete activity 2 – Clinician puts wet hand to child's face (3 attempts) 3 – Clinician puts wet hand to own face, and child then completes 4 – Child puts wet hand to face with auditory cue 5 – Child puts wet hand to face upon presentation.

Independence assessment

Jeni Malone

A carer questionnaire (Form 2.19) is used to establish the child's level of independence in feeding at home. This, along with observation of physical abilities, especially fine motor skills, and observation of EDS trials, is used to identify a child's developmental level in self-feeding. This is of great importance when setting EDS goals. In some cases a child has all the skills present to self-feed, and reasons for perceived lack of use of self-feeding need to be identified. Where refusal to self-feed is secondary to behavioural issues relating to food aversion, goals for improvement of self-feeding skills can be integrated early on in the setting of programme goals. Where a child is functioning at their fullest developmental level for self-feeding then priority is given to EDS goals. Placing an additional challenge of improving self-feeding would be too great a challenge for a child at this time and probably result in failure. Self-feeding issues in the context, for example, of physical limitations, can be addressed separately at a later stage or when appropriate.

The questionnaire also gives some indication of the feeding environment, routine and specific frustrations faced by carers. It may highlight issues such as an over-stimulating environment, for example a radio playing where auditory defensiveness is present, or inappropriate positioning for the child.

Medical assessment

When working with children with disabilities who present with EDS dysfunction, it is mandatory for the clinician to ensure a thorough medical assessment is conducted, either as part of the Fun with Food assessment process or preceding it. This ensures that the medical status of the child will not interfere with a successful outcome on the programme and that the child is not medically compromised. The doctor is requested specifically to address respiratory, neurological, physical, psychiatric and gastrointestinal issues. This includes medications and any impact they may have on swallow function or general alertness. The doctor is also requested to make any interventions they deem appropriate and which have not already been made, for example, investigations for gastro-oesophageal reflux and anti-reflux treatment. A paediatrician who knows the child already may be able to bypass most of this procedure. The doctor advises the team on the individual's medical stability and therefore eligibility for the programme.

Post-assessment

Carer Question & Answer time

The time is set aside for carers to ask questions and have them answered by the course co-ordinator. These typically include:

- 'When will I know if my child has a place?'
- 'What are the criteria for selection?'
- 'What if we cannot attend all the days?' and so on.

Assessment outcomes

- A summary of results is compiled in the Individual Assessment Summary (Form 2.20) and fed back to the carer.
- Interventions may be recommended by various clinicians that can be carried out by the carer prior to commencement on the programme; for example a sensory diet may be formulated between the carer and clinician.
- The team members meet to discuss and select candidates. A chart (Sample Candidate Summaries Form 2.21 on page 93) detailing summaries of the possible programme candidates may help in this process. The chart can be a simple summary of each part of the assessment process (eg represent the presence or absence of problems).
- Carers are informed of the offer of a place. For those for whom it is not appropriate, clear feedback on the reasons for this and an appropriate follow-up plan should be considered.
- At this time, specific goals for the programme for each child should be compiled so that they can be discussed with carers at programme commencement.
- Severity ratings are decided upon (see sample Form 2.22).
- Key-workers, who will work closely with the child and carer throughout the programme, are allocated, and this decision is made primarily on the needs basis. For example, a child with sensory issues may be allocated an occupational therapist as a key-worker, whereas a child with dominant nutritional issues may be allocated a dietitian as a key-worker. This is also, of course, resource dependent.

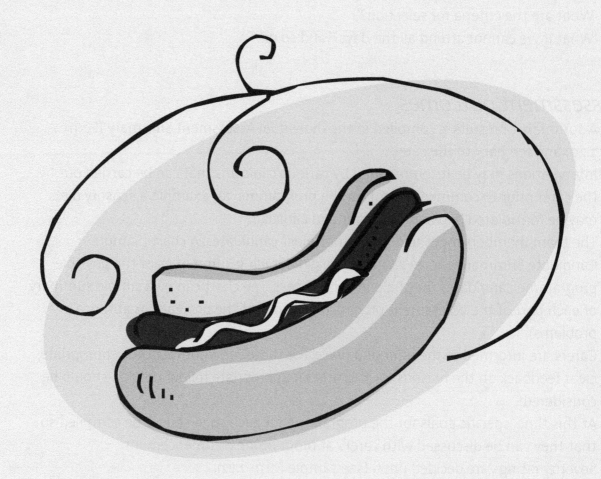

Chapter 2 Photocopiable master forms, records, diaries, questionnaires and sample forms

Form 2.1: Pre-assessment Case History Form

Name of client _____ Date of birth _____

Name of carer/carers _____

Relationship to child _____

Client's address _____

_____

_____

_____

Telephone _____ Mobile _____

Email _____

CONCERNS

Please outline your primary concerns regarding your child's eating and drinking:

_____

_____

_____

_____

_____

SERVICES

Please indicate what health or other professionals your child is involved with.

Current

Name			
Title			
Place of work			
Input provided			

Previous

Name			
Title			
Place of work			
Input provided			
When finished?			

Page 1 of 13

Form 2.1: *continued*

FEEDING HISTORY

Please outline what previous input your child has received with regard to eating & drinking from any health discipline, and the impact this has had on your child's eating & drinking skills.

_____

_____

_____

_____

_____

Any family history of eating & drinking/nutritional problems?   ☐ Yes   ☐ No
Please explain:

_____

_____

_____

_____

Tube feeding

History of tube feeding   ☐ Yes   ☐ No

Type of tube eg nasogastric/ PEG	Age at which inserted	Outcome	Still in use?		Age at which discontinued
_____	_____	_____	☐ Yes	☐ No	_____
_____	_____	_____	☐ Yes	☐ No	_____
_____	_____	_____	☐ Yes	☐ No	_____

Bottle/breast feeding

Identify which used and success/ease of use _____

_____

_____

Form 2.1: *continued*

Transitions

	Age	Ease of transition	Reason for success/failure
Breast			
Bottle			
Beaker/cup			
Purées			
Mash			
Lumpy foods (in other foods, eg beans)			
Separate lumps (eg bread, crisps)			

Thickeners

Has your child ever been prescribed thickeners?   ☐ Yes   ☐ No

Name the thickener prescribed _____

If used, why prescribed and did/does it make a difference?

_____

_____

Is your child still on thickeners?   ☐ Yes   ☐ No

Utensils

What utensils (for eating *and* drinking) does your child currently use and how appropriate for your child do you think they are?

For eating _____

_____

_____

For drinking _____

_____

_____

Form 2.1: *continued*

Strategies
What strategies to help your child's eating & drinking have you attempted previously?
Which have worked or not worked?

Worked _____

_____

Not worked _____

_____

BIRTH HISTORY

Pre-, peri- & postnatal history
Gestational age (in weeks) when born _____

Type of delivery _____

Length of stay in hospital _____

Identify any complications arising _____

_____

_____

MEDICAL HISTORY

Diagnosis(es) _____

_____

_____

Current health
General health _____

_____

Respiratory, eg history of broncho–pulmonary dysplasia, colds/pneumonia, chest or ear infections, allergies, aspiration.

_____

_____

Page 4 of 13

Form 2.1: *continued*

Gastrointestinal, eg history of reflux, constipation, or wind.

_____

_____

Neurological, eg history of epilepsy, learning or physical disability.

_____

_____

Hearing & Vision

_____

_____

Other

_____

_____

Medications

Drug name	Date prescribed	Outcome with use of medicine	Still in use?	
_____	_____	_____	☐ Yes	☐ No
_____	_____	_____	☐ Yes	☐ No
_____	_____	_____	☐ Yes	☐ No
_____	_____	_____	☐ Yes	☐ No
_____	_____	_____	☐ Yes	☐ No

Allergies

_____

Procedures

Investigation/Operation	Date	Outcome
_____	_____	_____
_____	_____	_____
_____	_____	_____

Form 2.1: *continued*

Sleep patterns

Sleeps whole night ☐ Yes ☐ No

If not, wakes how many times? _____

Is your child easy/difficult to settle? ☐ Easy ☐ Difficult

NUTRITIONAL HISTORY

Child's most recent weight _____

Measured by whom _____

On what date _____

Meat group

Does your child eat:

Meat	☐ Yes ☐ No	Fish	☐ Yes ☐ No
Cheese	☐ Yes ☐ No	Eggs	☐ Yes ☐ No

How often would your child eat these?

Twice daily ☐   Once daily ☐   Weekly ☐   Monthly ☐   Never ☐

Milk group

Does your child take:

Milk (eg formula, low-fat etc)	☐ Yes	☐ No
Cheese	☐ Yes	☐ No
Custards	☐ Yes	☐ No
Yoghurts	☐ Yes	☐ No
Milk puddings	☐ Yes	☐ No
Never	☐ Yes	☐ No

How much of these foods daily? _____

Do you add milk to your child's cereal? ☐ Yes ☐ No

Page 6 of 13

Form 2.1: *continued*

Fruit & Vegetable group

Does your child take fruit? ☐ Yes ☐ No

Does your child take vegetables? ☐ Yes ☐ No

What type? _____

How often?

Daily? ☐ Yes ☐ No   Weekly? ☐ Yes ☐ No

How many? _____

Potato & Cereal group

Does your child take cereal? ☐ Yes ☐ No

What type? _____

Does your child take bread? ☐ Yes ☐ No

What type?

Brown bread ☐ Yes ☐ No

White bread ☐ Yes ☐ No

Does your child take:

Potatoes ☐ Yes ☐ No   Rice ☐ Yes ☐ No

Pasta ☐ Yes ☐ No   Chips ☐ Yes ☐ No

Supplements

Has your child ever been prescribed nutritional supplements, high-energy sip drinks or milk shakes? ☐ Yes ☐ No

Supplement name	Date prescribed	Outcome with use	Still in use?
_____	_____	_____	☐ Yes ☐ No
_____	_____	_____	☐ Yes ☐ No
_____	_____	_____	☐ Yes ☐ No

If your child is currently tube fed, please identify the name of the feed precisely as it is on the label _____

Does your child take any remedies for constipation? ☐ Yes ☐ No

Please name them _____

Form 2.1: *continued*

EQUIPMENT

Wheelchair type and name _____

Home chair/school chair _____

Stander _____

Walker _____

Splints _____

Other _____

PHYSICAL/INDEPENDENCE

Please comment on your child's predominant tone/pattern, head control, sitting ability and general mobility if appropriate _____

_____

_____

Upper limb function

Is there a problem with how your child uses their hands? If yes state if there is a preference, and for which hand _____

Is reaching/grasping possible? ☐ Yes ☐ No

Positioning

Identify the usual positioning for feeding at home _____
Identify the usual position for feeding at school/centre _____

Self-feeding

Does your child feed himself/herself? ☐ Yes ☐ No
If yes, how successful is this? _____

Page 8 of 13

Form 2.1: *continued*

Play

Does your child avoid or seek out:

Messy play	☐ Avoid	☐ Seek out
Playground equipment	☐ Avoid	☐ Seek out
Moving toys	☐ Avoid	☐ Seek out

Does your child prefer: ☐ sedentary play ☐ to be always 'on the go' *(active)*

Identify preferred toys _____

_____

_____

FEEDING ENVIRONMENT

Feeders

If not an independent feeder please identify:

Home:	Main feeder	Other feeder	Child's preferred feeder
	_____	_____	_____
School/Centre:	Main feeder	Other feeder	Child's preferred feeder
	_____	_____	_____

Other (identify situation) _____

	Main feeder	Other feeder	Child's preferred feeder
	_____	_____	_____

Environments

Describe environments, eg noisy/quiet, number of people, seating arrangements, etc

Home _____

_____

School/Centre _____

_____

Other _____

_____

Form 2.1: *continued*

<table>
<tr><td align="center">ORAL MOTOR</td></tr>
</table>

ENT

Is there a family history of ear, nose and throat (ENT) problems? ☐ Yes ☐ No

Identify _____

Does your child have a history of, or current ENT problems? ☐ Yes ☐ No

Identify _____

Dentition

What teeth have emerged? ☐ First set *(baby)* ☐ Second set *(adult)*

If first set, which ones and how many? _____

Saliva control

Does your child drool/dribble? ☐ Yes ☐ No

Rate its severity ☐ Mild ☐ Moderate ☐ Severe

How many times a day would you:

Wipe face _____ Change bib _____ Change clothes _____

Have you tried any strategies to help control drooling? ☐ Yes ☐ No

Identify _____

Mouth

Do your child's jaws, mouth, tongue, lips function properly as far as you

can see? ☐ Yes ☐ No

Identify particular issues you have in this area _____

Page 10 of 13

Form 2.1: *continued*

Non-nutritive

Does your child use a dummy/soother   ☐ Yes   ☐ No

With what frequency during the day:

    ☐ At night only   ☐ Occasionally   ☐ Frequently   ☐ Always in mouth

Does your child place in his mouth:

Hands	☐ Never	☐ Occasionally	☐ Frequently	☐ Always
Toys	☐ Never	☐ Occasionally	☐ Frequently	☐ Always
Finger foods	☐ Never	☐ Occasionally	☐ Frequently	☐ Always

Oral habits

Identify those habits your child has a history of, or currently exhibits

Note which is dominant and how frequently engaged in *(eg thumb/finger sucking, tongue thrusting, teeth grinding, lip biting/sucking/licking, mouth breathing, snoring)*

_____

_____

Coughing, Choking & Gagging

Can your child cough?   ☐ Yes   ☐ No

During eating and drinking, does your child:

Cough	☐ Never	☐ Occasionally	☐ Frequently	☐ Always
Choke	☐ Never	☐ Occasionally	☐ Frequently	☐ Always
Gag	☐ Never	☐ Occasionally	☐ Frequently	☐ Always

Is this more noticeable for: ☐ Liquids   ☐ Solids   ☐ Lumpy foods   ☐ All

Face & head activities

How does your child respond to:

Face washing _____

Teeth brushing _____

Hair brushing _____

Form 2.1: *continued*

Is your child sensitive to temperatures around the face or in the mouth?   ☐ Yes   ☐ No

Is there a history of oral injury/invasive procedures in the oral area?   ☐ Yes   ☐ No

Please identify these _____

Speech

Does your child use *(tick which applies)*:   ☐ vowels   ☐ consonants
                                                  ☐ words   ☐ sentences

Is your child's speech clearly understood?   ☐ Yes   ☐ No

Communication/behaviour

How does your child communicate generally? _____

_____

How is your child's behaviour generally? _____

_____

How is your child's behaviour around eating & drinking? _____

_____

Identify the behaviours you are concerned about _____

_____

_____

How does your child react to change/new situations/places? _____

_____

Comment on attention during feeding. Are distractions used? What? Why?

_____

Does your child show hunger?   ☐ Yes   ☐ No

How? _____

_____

Form 2.1: *continued*

Does your child have preferred food & drinks?   ☐ Yes   ☐ No
Identify _____

_____

Does your child have non-preferred food & drinks?   ☐ Yes   ☐ No
Identify _____

_____

How often do you attempt to introduce non-preferred items?
    ☐ Each meal   ☐ Daily   ☐ Weekly   ☐ Monthly   ☐ Infrequently   ☐ Never
How does your child signal 'like' regarding food & drink items?

_____

How does your child signal dislike regarding food & drink items?

_____

How is your child's behaviour/mood, and does it show change:
Before meals _____
During meals _____
After meals _____
How does your child respond at the start of meals? _____

_____

How does your child respond to changes in eating & drinking? _____

_____

Other comments:

Form 2.2: Pre-assessment Sample Food Diary

Name of child __David Power__ Day _____ Date __8th February__ Friday

Time fed	Location/ Seating used	Food/Drink descriptions	Amount offered	Amount taken	Who fed the child	How long did it take?	Outcome
7.00 a.m.	In Mum's bed	Bottle of SMA progress	8ozs/236ml	Nil – was sick	David himself	15 minutes	Vomited all up
9.30 a.m.	In the kitchen in his high chair	Thin porridge with full cream milk	2ozs/56g of porridge & 4ozs/118ml milk	About half	Mum with David helping	30 minutes	Fine
10.30 a.m.	Around the house while playing	Blackcurrant drink & 2 scoops of thickening agent	4ozs/118ml	All	David	On and off until lunch time	Fine
12.00 noon	In the kitchen in his high chair	Jar of chicken & vegetable dinner – 4 months. 1 yoghurt	4oz/112g jar & 2oz/56g pot of yoghurt	None of the dinner and all of the yoghurt	Mum	40 minutes	A lot on bib
1.00 p.m.	In his bed	Bottle of SMA progress	8ozs/236ml	All	David	15 minutes	
3.30 p.m.	In the main room watching television	Blackcurrant drink & 2 scoops thickening agents & chocolate biscuits	4ozs/118ml of drink & 2 biscuits	All the drink and both biscuits	David	On and off until dinner time.	Vomited up half
6.00 p.m.	In the kitchen in his high chair	Burger cut up, mashed potatoes & puréed peas	1 burger, 3 tbls of potatoes & 1 tsp of peas	None of the burger or potato. 2 tsp of peas	Mum and older sister	1 hour	Fine
7.30 p.m.	In his bed	Bottle of SMA progress	8ozs/236ml	6ozs/170ml (fell asleep)	David	15 minutes	Fine Was irritable through night

Form 2.3: Daily Food Diary

Name of child _____ Day _____ Date _____

Time fed	Location/ Seating used	Food/Drink descriptions	Amount offered	Amount taken	Who fed the child	How long did it take?	Outcome

* Please say if food is puréed, cut up or mashed, and if drinks are thickened with a thickening agent. Use everyday measures such as teaspoons or cupfuls if preferable

Form 2.4: Video of Eating & Drinking Session Permission Form

Please find enclosed a Video Permission Form which you are required to sign and bring with you on assessment day. The aim of videotaping is to obtain a video record of your child's eating & drinking & swallowing skills and the interaction around mealtime. Videotaping is an integral part of the Fun with Food programme and will happen at various points along the way.

Name of child _____

Address _____

_____

_____

_____

Date of Birth _____

Date _____

I hereby give consent to the Fun with Food programme to videotape my child and their carers for the duration of the programme. I understand the tapes will be used for assessment, therapy and monitoring purposes.

Signed _____ (Carer of child)

Relationship to child _____

Form 2.5: Carer Construction of
Eating & Drinking & Swallowing Problem

Name of child _____   Date _____

1   What are your concerns regarding your child's feeding development? Please outline
    them below.

    _____

    _____

    _____

2   Identify other people's comments regarding your child's EDS problems (including
    siblings, grandparents etc).

    _____

    _____

    _____

3   What are your expectations for your child's development in this area without
    intervention?

    _____

    _____

    _____

4   If your child is accepted onto the Fun with Food programme, what do you expect to
    gain from the programme for both your child and yourself?

    _____

    _____

    _____

Form 2.5: *continued*

5 How would you summarise your child's eating & drinking problem?

_____

_____

_____

6 Would you agree if someone said your child's eating problem was related to behaviour, either in some part or totally?

_____

_____

_____

7 Are you willing to attend all the days of the programme?

☐ Yes   ☐ No

Your answer will affect your child being accepted onto the course.

8 Who will be able to attend every day with your child?

Name _____   Relationship _____

Name _____   Relationship _____

Name _____   Relationship _____

9 Please rate your child's EDS difficulty on the scale on the next sheet.

Tick or circle the box on each row which most represents your child's eating behaviour.

Signed _____

Form 2.5: continued

Please tick or circle the box on each row which most represents your child's eating behaviour.

	1	2	3	4	5
Food approach behaviour	He/she will sit easily at the table	Occasionally he/she will be difficult to sit at the table, or leave early	Frequently he/she will be difficult to sit at the table, or will be in & out of his chair or leave early	Sometimes will sit, but it always takes a lot of effort and will be in & out of the chair all the time	He/she will not go near a table or place where food also is present
Time spent eating	Will eat like other children interspersed with chatting and fun	Takes a number of bites/drinks but not as much as I would like	Will take bites or sips but I can count on two hands the number of times this happens during a meal	Will eat or drink very rarely and it is effortful for him/her. He/she spends more time thinking about eating than actually doing it	Will not eat or drink at all
Eating & Drinking – range etc	no problems – eats and drinks almost everything offered – like other children really	some minor problems – he occasionally refuses specific items of food or drink	He gets by but I have to plan what I can give him/her for every meal. Refuses a lot of foods/drinks but it is not impossible to feed, or to go out with	A lot of problems with food. Although he/she will eat or drink something, it is limited and I have difficulty planning for him/her	Won't eat or drink at all, won't even touch or smell food or let anything near mouth or face like teeth brushing or face washing
Sensory/tactile/ of daily living responses	Just like other kids with regard to teeth brushing, washing hands, face washing, hair brushing etc	Doesn't like things like teeth brushing, face washing but does it daily	Doesn't like these. I can do these activities some days but not all by any means, and it is an effort	Hates things like teeth brushing, face washing or getting hands dirty. Occasionally, it can get done – once a week maybe but it is difficult	Won't let you touch activities his/her face, mouth or hands at all
Behavioural reactions	Doesn't react big time to food or drink. You wouldn't notice it	Will comment or turn away occasionally but really he/she gets on with it without too much fuss	Shows obvious dislike at every meal but despite this generally will attempt eating	Will scream, cry, etc but will not run away or turn away physically from food or drink	Screams, runs away when food mentioned. You couldn't put him/her in the same room as food. Gets sick
How much time/work I have to do to get my child to eat – effects	No time greater than for other kids	A little encouragement is needed and I will have to work out something different for him/her sometimes	Needs a lot of thought and I have to prepare especially for him/her but it is doable.	Affects my life considerably. Requires a lot of thought and effort but doesn't totally take over	A lot of time preparing, finding the right food or drink that he/she will eat, coercing him/her to actually eat. My day revolves around it

Form 2.6: Food Approach Behaviour Form

Name of child _____   Therapist _____   Date _____

Food Approach Behaviour *Behaviours based on per cent of time behaviour observed during activity*	Preferred & Non-preferred foods	Length of time in seconds	Less than 19%	20–39%	40–59%	60–79%	Greater than 80%
TOTAL TIME							
APPROACH BEHAVIOUR: Sit with ease	Time: preferred foods						
	Time: non-preferred foods						
APPROACH BEHAVIOUR: Actual eating	Time: preferred foods						
	Time: non-preferred foods						

Form 2.7: Oral-Nutritional Behaviour Form

Name of child _____   Therapist _____   Date _____

Oral-nutritional behaviour _Behaviours based on incidence / frequency count_	Number of contacts Preferred foods	Number of contacts Non-preferred foods	Never	Sometimes	Occasionally	Frequently	Constantly
Non-oral contact							
Pre-oral contact							
Intraoral contact							
Pharyngeal contact							

Form 2.8: Flavours & Consistencies Record

Name of child _____ Therapist _____ Date _____

Food range	Number of spoons/sips taken	Never	Sometimes	Occasionally	Frequently	Constantly
Flavours/Tastes						
Bland food						
Savoury food						
Sweet food						
Spicy food						
Bitter food						
Consistencies/Textures						
Liquid						
Purée						
Mash						
Roughly mashed						
Mixed texture						
Soft separate lumps						
Hard separate lumps						

Never = behaviour did not occur during videotape

Sometimes = behaviour observed 1–2 times

Occasionally = behaviour observed 3–5 times

Frequently = behaviour observed 5–9 times

Constantly = behaviour observed 10+ times

Form 2.9: EDS Script

TOTAL VIDEO TIME _____

Name of child _____   Date _____

Page No _____   Therapist _____

Speaker	Statement	Notes

Form 2.10: EDS Script Summary Count

Name of child _____   Date _____

Therapist _____

Area	Carer 1:	Carer 2:	Child:
Words in total per individual			
% of total words by all communication partners			
No. utterances in total			
% of total words by all communication partners			
No. utterances related to food			
% of individual's total			
No. negative utterances			
% of individual's total			
No. repetitions of own utterances			
% of individual's total			
No. repetitions of child's utterances			
% of individual's total			
No. praise/reinforcing utterances			
% of individual's total			
No. questions used			
% of individual's total			
No. directions re food			
% of individual's total			
No. positive utterances			
% of individual's total			
No. negotiations			
% of individual's total			
Length of tape = _____ minutes _____ seconds	wpm	wpm	wpm
No. words per minute of videotape – wpm =			

Form 2.11: Sample Carer–Child Interaction Summary Form

Person & Name	Constructive behaviour	Non-constructive behaviour
Carer 1	Models eating Uses praise	Asks the child why he doesn't like food Constantly urging the child to eat
Carer 2	Smiles	Gives no feedback to the child Arms folded
Child	Sits at table initially	Throws plate Turns away from the table Makes self sick

Signed (by clinician) _____

Form 2.12: Carer–Child Interaction Summary Form

Person & Name	Constructive behaviour	Non-constructive behaviour
Carer 1		
Carer 2		
Child		

Signed (by clinician) _____

Form 2.13: Nutritional Intake Form

Name of child _____ Date _____

Clinician _____

Area	Date 1	Date 2	Date 3	Date 4	Date 5
Weight					
Height					
Energy intake					
Protein intake					
Calcium intake					
Iron intake					
Vitamin C intake					
Vitamin D intake					

NOTES

Calculation guidelines

Energy intake relative to height, age, sex & physical impairment

Protein intake relative to age, sex & current weight (kg) x protein requirement for height age per kg body weight

Calcium, iron, Vitamins C & D intake relative to chronological age and sex

Ratings: 1 = very low, 2 = low, 3 = normal, 4 = high, 5 = very high

Based on Krick et al, 1996 & Cocks, 2000

Form 2.14: Tastes & Textures Questionnaire

Thank you for completing this questionnaire.

1   When listing the foods that you have tried or that your child likes, remember to include fruit, vegetables, meat, fish, eggs and dairy products (eg yoghurts, cheese), ice-cream and also other desserts.

2   When describing the food consistencies, use the following as a guide:

Purée: (with no lumps)

   (a)   A smooth pouring uniform consistency, eg tinned tomato soup or thin custard

   (b)   A smooth uniform consistency that drops rather than pours from a spoon and cannot be eaten with a fork, eg thick custard

   (c)   A thick smooth uniform consistency that holds its shape on a plate and can be eaten with a spoon or a fork, eg a mousse.

Mash: (with no lumps)

Roughly mashed: (small lumps with the mash)

Soft separate lumps: (eg small finely chopped pieces of cooked carrot, sausage and banana separate from other food on the plate)

Mixed textures: (eg baked beans where there are beans + sauce, minestrone soup with soup + pasta pieces)

Hard lumps: (eg small pieces of raw carrot or apple).

3   When describing the consistencies of the drinks, use the following as a guide:

Liquid: (eg water or juice)

Thicker liquid: This leaves a thin coating on the back of a spoon (eg milk shakes)

Medium thick liquid: This leaves a thick coating on the back of a spoon (eg ordinary juice, water or squash thickened with a thickening agent to a syrup consistency)

Thick liquid: (eg ordinary juice, squash or lemonade/soda which is thickened with a thickening agent to a pouring custard consistency).

4   When completing information about a food or drink, always name it. For example:

Food 1. (name it) Apple   Consistency: Purée (no lumps)

Page 1 of 5

Form 2.14: *continued*

Name of child _____ Carer _____
Clinician _____ Date _____

1 List all the foods that your child likes and how frequently they are taken.

Food 1. (name it) _____ Consistency _____
How often is the food taken?
Monthly ☐ Weekly ☐ 2 times a week ☐ 3–5 times a week ☐ Daily ☐

Food 2. (name it) _____ Consistency _____
How often is the food taken?
Monthly ☐ Weekly ☐ 2 times a week ☐ 3–5 times a week ☐ Daily ☐

Food 3. (name it) _____ Consistency _____
How often is the food taken?
Monthly ☐ Weekly ☐ 2 times a week ☐ 3–5 times a week ☐ Daily ☐

Food 4. (name it) _____ Consistency _____
How frequently is the food taken?
Monthly ☐ Weekly ☐ 2 times a week ☐ 3–5 times a week ☐ Daily ☐

Food 5. (name it) _____ Consistency _____
How frequently is the food taken?
Monthly ☐ Weekly ☐ 2 times a week ☐ 3–5 times a week ☐ Daily ☐

Others:
For any other food, please list and provide the information that you have given for foods 1–5.
Food (name it) _____ Consistency _____
How frequently is the food taken?
Monthly ☐ Weekly ☐ 2 times a week ☐ 3–5 times a week ☐ Daily ☐

Form 2.14: *continued*

Food (name it) _____ Consistency _____

How frequently is the food taken?

Monthly ☐   Weekly ☐   2 times a week ☐   3–5 times a week ☐   Daily ☐

2 List all the drinks that your child likes and how frequently they are taken.

Drink 1. (name it) _____ Consistency _____

How often is it taken?

Monthly ☐   Weekly ☐   2 times a week ☐   3–5 times a week ☐   Daily ☐

Drink 2. (name it) _____ Consistency _____

How often is it taken?

Monthly ☐   Weekly ☐   2 times a week ☐   3–5 times a week ☐   Daily ☐

Drink 3. (name it) _____ Consistency _____

How often is it taken?

Monthly ☐   Weekly ☐   2 times a week ☐   3–5 times a week ☐   Daily ☐

Drink 4. (name it) _____ Consistency _____

How often is it taken?

Monthly ☐   Weekly ☐   2 times a week ☐   3–5 times a week ☐   Daily ☐

Drink 5. (name it) _____ Consistency _____

How often is it taken?

Monthly ☐   Weekly ☐   2 times a week ☐   3–5 times a week ☐   Daily ☐

Form 2.14: *continued*

3 What food consistencies would you avoid giving your child? Please tick in the boxes those that apply.

Purée (no lumps) ☐

Mash (no lumps) ☐

Roughly mashed (small lumps in with the mash) ☐

Soft separate lumps (eg cooked carrots, banana, pear or sausage) ☐

Hard lumps (eg apple or raw carrot) ☐

Why do you avoid these consistencies?

_____

_____

_____

_____

4 What drink consistencies would you avoid giving your child? Please tick in the boxes those that apply.

Liquid (eg water or squash) ☐

Medium thick liquids (eg Calpol® consistency) ☐

Thick consistencies (eg pouring custard consistency) ☐

Why do you avoid these consistencies?

_____

_____

_____

_____

5 Tick the flavours that your child likes and give examples of the foods.

Salty ☐   Sour ☐   Spicy ☐

Sweet ☐   Bitter ☐

Form 2.14: *continued*

6 Does your child react negatively to any of the following? Tick the boxes as
appropriate. Describe the reaction.

Smell of food and drink	☐	_____
Sound of food and drink being prepared	☐	_____
Other people's food and drink	☐	_____
Touching food and drink utensils	☐	_____
Temperature of food and drink	☐	_____

7 List three foods that you and the person who will attend with you really like:

Food 1. _____

Food 2. _____

Food 3. _____

8 List three foods that you and the person who will attend with you really dislike:

Food 1. _____

Food 2. _____

Food 3. _____

Form 2.15: Oral Motor Exam (OME) Form 1

Name of child _____ Therapist _____ Date _____

Oral structure	Observe structure at rest	Position and movement pattern Non-nutritive	Position and movement pattern Nutritive 1: Eating	Position and movement pattern Nutritive 2: Drinking
Lips	Open ☐ Closed ☐ Retracted ☐	Kiss and hold ☐ Smile posture ☐ Puff cheeks & maintain seal ☐ Spatula between lips ☐ Blow bubbles (lip rounding) ☐	Open ☐ Closed ☐ Limited movement ☐ Sucking or suckling movement ☐ Active use ☐ Loss of food ☐ Awareness ☐	Efficient lip closure: Cup ☐ Straw ☐ Poor lip seal ☐ Loss of fluid ☐ Awareness ☐
Jaw & Teeth	Symmetry: ☐ Normal ☐ Deviation left ☐ Deviation right ☐ Jaw grinding ☐ Jaw clenching Mandible: Protruded/Retracted Maxilla: Protruded/Retracted Occlusion: Normal ☐ Crossbite ☐ Underbite ☐ Overbite ☐ Open bite ☐	Open and close jaw ☐ Clatter teeth (3 times) ☐ Chewy Tube®: ☐ Bite and hold ☐ Chewing ☐ Number of cycles Preferred side for chewing _____	Suckling and sucking movement ☐ Munching pattern ☐ Components of diagonal rotary movement ☐ Co-ordinated rotary movement ☐ Co-ordinated circular rotary movement ☐ Preferred side for chewing/not :	Wide excursions ☐ Bite onto cup/straw ☐ Graded jaw movement ☐

Form 2.15: *continued*

Oral structure	Observe structure at rest	Position and movement pattern Non-nutritive	Position and movement pattern Nutritive 1: Eating	Position and movement pattern Nutritive 2: Drinking
Jaw & Teeth (continued)	Teeth: Condition (gums, cavities, decay etc) Arrangement: ☐ Normal ☐ Missing teeth ☐ Misaligned Hygiene: ☐ Good ☐ Poor		☐ Used in biting ☐ Used in chewing	
Tongue	Position: ☐ Normal ☐ Protruded ☐ Retracted Frenulum: ☐ Normal ☐ Short	Stick out tongue: Midline ☐ Deviation L Deviation R Elevation: Yes/No Tongue-tip down: Yes/No Side to side: Yes/No/Limited Range of motion (ROM)	Chewing: Up-down movement ☐ Anterior/Posterior movement ☐ Able to form bolus ☐ Lateralisation of bolus ☐ Move food across midline ☐ Tongue-tip elevation ☐ Swallow: Normal ☐ Anterior/Posterior movement ☐ Tongue pumping ☐ Delayed movement ☐	Position: Inside mouth ☐ Under cup ☐ Under straw ☐ Movement: Front/Back ☐ Up/down ☐ Elevated ☐

Page 2 of 3

Form 2.15: continued

Oral structure	Observe structure at rest	Position and movement pattern Non-nutritive	Position and movement pattern Nutritive 1: Eating	Position and movement pattern Nutritive 2: Drinking
Palate & Pharynx	Palate height: ☐ Normal ☐ High ☐ Low width: ☐ Normal ☐ Narrow ☐ Wide Colour: Normal/Abnormal Tonsils: Present/removed/enlarged	Phonation of 'ah' Movement: ☐ Symmetrical ☐ Weakness Left ☐ Weakness Right ☐ Uncertain Coughing: Yes/No/ Not observed Gag reflex: ☐ Normal ☐ Absent ☐ Hypersensitive ☐ Hyposensitive	Suck–Swallow–Breathe Co-ordination: ☐ Difficulty to co-ordinate ☐ Some coughing and choking ☐ Well co-ordinated Reflexes: ☐ Gag reflex ☐ Cough reflex ☐ Swallow reflex Other: _____	
Safety	Oral motor skills observed support safe eating and drinking: Yes/No			

Page 3 of 3

Form 2.16: Oral Motor Exam (OME) Form 2

Name of child _____   Date _____

Clinician _____

1. Oral structures at rest

Face	☐ Symmetrical	☐ Asymmetrical		
Tone	☐ Normal	☐ Low	☐ High	☐ Fluctuating
Mandible	Position:	☐ Normal	☐ Low	☐ High

Appearance _____

Lips	☐ Open	☐ Closed		
Drooling	☐ Absent	☐ Mild	☐ Moderate	☐ Severe
Teeth	☐ Primary	☐ Mixed	☐ Adult	

Condition _____

Tongue	Position:	☐ Normal	☐ Protruded	☐ Retracted
Palate	☐ Normal	☐ Narrow	☐ High	☐ Other

If other, please describe _____

_____

_____

2. Sensation

(a) Face

Tolerates:

Deep pressure/massage cream on face	☐ Yes	☐ No
Deep pressure to temporo-mandibular joint	☐ Yes	☐ No
Deep pressure around mouth	☐ Yes	☐ No
Deep pressure on lips	☐ Yes	☐ No
Touch on face with	☐ Fingers	☐ Puppet ☐ Other

Form 2.16: *continued*

(b) Oral

Tolerates stimulation to:

Gums/teeth	☐ Yes	☐ No
Inside of cheeks	☐ Yes	☐ No
Tongue blade	☐ Yes	☐ No
Lateral tongue margins	☐ Yes	☐ No
Alveolar ridge	☐ Yes	☐ No
Palate	☐ Yes	☐ No

Tool used :   ☐ Finger ☐ Toothette ☐ Infadent ☐ Vibrating Toothette ☐ NUK®

(c) Gag

☐ Present   ☐ absent

Where elicited _____

3. Oral imitation

(a) Jaw

Slowly open jaw (hold 3–5 seconds)	☐ Yes	☐ No	☐ Uncertain
Slowly close jaw	☐ Yes	☐ No	☐ Uncertain
Clatter teeth (3 or more repetitions)	☐ Yes	☐ No	☐ Uncertain

Comments _____

(b) Lips

Kiss and hold	☐ Yes	☐ No	☐ Uncertain
Smile	☐ Yes	☐ No	☐ Uncertain
Puff cheeks and maintain seal	☐ Yes	☐ No	☐ Uncertain

Rapid movements

Alternate smile & kiss postures ☐ WNL ☐ Slow ☐ Unco-ordinated
                                 ☐ Uncertain

(Pa Pa Pa) ☐ WNL ☐ Slow ☐ Unco-ordinated
            ☐ Uncertain

Page 2 of 6

Form 2.16: *continued*

(c) Palate

Elevation (Phonation of 'ah')   ☐ Symmetrical   ☐ Weakness Left
                                 ☐ Uncertain   ☐ Weakness Right

(d) Tongue

Protruded tongue   ☐ Midline   ☐ Deviation Left   ☐ Deviation Right   ☐ Uncertain

Side to side   ☐ Yes   ☐ Limited movement   ☐ Uncertain

Elevation   ☐ Yes   ☐ No   ☐ Uncertain

Rapid movements

t – t – t   ☐ Within normal limits   ☐ Slow   ☐ Unco-ordinated   ☐ Uncertain

k – k – k   ☐ WNL   ☐ Slow   ☐ Unco-ordinated   ☐ Uncertain

t – k – t   ☐ WNL   ☐ Slow   ☐ Unco-ordinated   ☐ Uncertain

4. Oral motor activities

(a) Whistle/Horn

Lip closure	☐ Yes	☐ No	☐ Uncertain
Tongue retraction	☐ Yes	☐ No	☐ Uncertain
Breath support	☐ Yes	☐ No	☐ Uncertain
Jaw stability present	☐ Yes	☐ No	☐ Uncertain

(b) Straw

Lip seal	☐ Yes	☐ No	☐ Uncertain
Jaw stability	☐ Yes	☐ No	☐ Uncertain
Tongue retraction	☐ Yes	☐ No	☐ Uncertain
Lip rounding	☐ Yes	☐ No	☐ Uncertain

(c) Bubbles

Lip rounding	☐ Yes	☐ No	☐ Uncertain
Grading airflow	☐ Yes	☐ No	☐ Uncertain
Jaw stability	☐ Yes	☐ No	☐ Uncertain

Form 2.16: *continued*

(d) Chewy Tube

Bite & hold	☐ Yes	☐ No	☐ Uncertain
Chewing	☐ Yes	☐ No	☐ Uncertain
Number of cycles	_____		

(e) Spatula

Lip closure	☐ Yes	☐ No	☐ Uncertain
Lip strength	☐ Yes	☐ No	☐ Uncertain
Jaw stability	☐ Yes	☐ No	☐ Uncertain
Lip–jaw dissociation	☐ Yes	☐ No	☐ Uncertain

5. Eating

(a) Note method/s of intake _____

(b) Non-chewing tasks

Jaw _____

Lips _____

Tongue _____

Loss of food _____

Awareness _____

(c) Chewing tasks

Jaw _____

Preferred side of chewing _____

Lips	☐ Open	☐ Closed	
	☐ Loss of food	☐ Awareness	
Tongue	☐ Able to form a bolus		
	☐ Lateralisation		
	☐ Move across midline		
Stage of chewing	☐ Munching	☐ Diagonal	☐ Rotary

Form 2.16: *continued*

(d) Swallow   ☐ Normal   ☐ Delayed   ☐ Multiple

☐ At risk of aspiration. Identify why _____

Results of swallow studies _____

Dependent on consistencies _____

6. Drinking

(a) Method of intake _____

(b) Oral functions during drinking

Jaw _____

Lips _____

Tongue _____

(c) Liquid management

Retrieval: ☐ Single sip   ☐ Series of single sips

Co-ordinated with swallow and breathing?   ☐ Yes   ☐ No

Swallow: ☐ Single   ☐ Multiple   ☐ Delayed   ☐ Coughing   ☐ Choking

Comments _____

7. Speech

(a) Child communicates   ☐ Verbally   ☐ Non-verbally

Describe _____

_____

(b) Associated movement of body & head   ☐ Yes   ☐ No

(c) Jaw movement during speech

Words	☐ Graded	☐ Co-ordinated	☐ Symmetrical
Sentences	☐ Graded	☐ Co-ordinated	☐ Symmetrical
Song	☐ Graded	☐ Co-ordinated	☐ Symmetrical

Page 5 of 6

Form 2.16: *continued*

(d) Lip movement ☐ Graded ☐ Co-ordinated ☐ Symmetrical
  Words ☐ Graded ☐ Co-ordinated ☐ Symmetrical
  Sentences ☐ Graded ☐ Co-ordinated ☐ Symmetrical
  Song ☐ Graded ☐ Co-ordinated ☐ Symmetrical

(e) Tongue movement ☐ Graded ☐ Co-ordinated ☐ Symmetrical
  Words ☐ Graded ☐ Co-ordinated ☐ Symmetrical
  Sentences ☐ Graded ☐ Co-ordinated ☐ Symmetrical
  Song ☐ Graded ☐ Co-ordinated ☐ Symmetrical

(f) Production of bilabial sounds ☐ Yes ☐ No

(g) Production of alveolar sounds ☐ Yes ☐ No

(h) Production of velar sounds ☐ Yes ☐ No

(i) Production of vowels (lip rounding) ☐ Adequate ☐ Limited ☐ Poor

(j) Clarity of speech ☐ Good ☐ Poor ☐ Uncertain
Describe _____

Form 2:17: Summary Oral Motor Exam (OME) Form

Name of child _____ Date _____

Clinician _____

Area	Notes
At rest	
Sensory system	
Oral imitation	
Oral motor activities	
Eating & drinking functions	
Swallow function	
Programme recommendations Oral awareness	
Normalisation to touch	
Oral exploration	
Oral motor activities	

Signed _____

Form 2.18 Sensory Assessment

Name of child _____ Date _____

Clinician _____

Activity	1 Did not complete	2 Assumes position	3 On 3rd attempt	4 On 2nd attempt	5 On 1st attempt
Vestibular					
Linear – up/down					
Orientation – prone/upright					
Rotary – spin					

Key 1 below gives details of parameters for this chart

Key 1: 1. Child did not complete activity
2. Child assumes position
3. Child completes activity on third presentation/attempt
4. Child completes activity on second presentation/attempt
5. Child completes activity on first presentation/attempt

Key 2 refers to the information on page 89

Key 2: 1. Child did not complete activity
2. Therapist-led activity – ie therapist completes activity on child
3. Therapist models behaviour and child completes activity
4. Child completes activity with auditory cue
5. Child completes activity upon presentation

Form 2.18: *continued*

Activity	1 Did not complete	2 Therapist led	3 Behaviour modelled	4 Auditory cue	5 Completed activity
Tactile Processing – Haptic/Facial					
Gritty – sand → hands					
Sticky – putty → hands					
Soft/fluffy → hands					
Soft/fluffy → face					
Vibration → hands					
Vibration → face					
Wet/liquid – paint → hands					
Wet/liquid – water → hands/arms					
Wet/liquid – water → face					
Dry/rubbing – towel → hands/arms					
Dry/rubbing – towel → face					
Deep pressure/massage – cream → hands/arms					
Deep pressure/massage – cream → face					
Deep pressure – TMJ → mouth					
Rotary deep pressure – TMJ → mouth					
Deep pressure → around mouth					
Deep pressure → lips					
Tactile Processing – Oral					
Deep pressure/stroking → gums					
Deep pressure → cheek walls					
Deep pressure → tongue					
Deep pressure → palate					
Olfaction					
Sweet					
Savoury					

Key 2 on page 1 of this Form gives details of parameters for this chart

Page 2 of 2

Form 2.19: Independence Questionnaire

Name of child _____ Date _____

Carer _____ Clinician _____

Please tick

1 How is your child normally positioned to have his meals?

☐ Sitting on regular chair at kitchen table

☐ Sitting in own supportive seat at kitchen table

☐ Sitting in own supportive seat with tray

☐ Sitting on floor

☐ Sitting on couch/armchair

☐ Other (please specify) _____

2 If your child uses a specialised supportive seat please state name of seat/chair

_____

3 Which of the following best describes a regular meal with your child?

Child:

☐ is fed whole meal

☐ finger feeds some of meal

☐ finger feeds all of meal

☐ spoon feeds some of meal with hand-over-hand assistance

☐ spoon feeds some of meal independently

☐ spoon feeds all of meal independently

☐ uses spoon and fork

☐ uses knife and fork

☐ uses bottle with assistance

☐ uses bottle independently

☐ uses beaker/cup with assistance

☐ uses beaker/cup independently (including replacing on table)

☐ other (please specify) _____

Page 1 of 3

Form 2.19: *continued*

4 If your child finger feeds, what food items will he/she accept (please list)?

_____

_____

5 If your child has specific cutlery or utensils please state name or type (eg small plastic spoon, plastic beaker with handles)

_____

_____

6 When helping your child develop self-feeding skills, what do you find difficult to cope with?

☐ The mess involved
☐ Not having the time needed
☐ Too many distractions
☐ You don't like food yourself
☐ Frustration at poor progress
☐ Conflict with other adults over behaviour
☐ Child's behaviour
☐ None
☐ Other (please specify)

7 Who else is normally present at mealtimes in your home?

☐ Other carer/carer (please specify)

_____

☐ Siblings (include ages)

_____

☐ Other (please specify)

_____

Form 2.19: *continued*

8 Which of the following distractions might happen at a typical mealtime?

☐ TV left on

☐ Radio/music on

☐ People coming and going from table

☐ Other children needing attention

☐ None

☐ Other (please explain) _____

Form 2.20: Individual Assessment Summary

Name of child _____ Date _____

Medical diagnoses

1 _____

2 _____

3 _____

Identify carer concerns

1 _____

2 _____

3 _____

Area	Summary	Therapist
Food approach behaviours		
Carer–Child interaction		
Nutrition		
Tastes & Textures		
Oral motor		
Sensory processing		
Independence		
Medical		

Page 1 of 2

Form 2.20: *continued*

EDS aversion details

Is EDS aversion present? ☐ Yes ☐ No

If so is it ...? ☐ Total ☐ Selective

Identify specifics of EDS aversion 1 _____

2 _____

3 _____

Identify possible causes of/
contributors to EDS aversion 1 _____

2 _____

3 _____

Estimate severity of EDS aversion ☐ Not present ☐ Mild ☐ Moderate ☐ Severe ☐ Profound

Fun with Food candidacy

Is this child a candidate for Fun with Food programme ? ☐ Yes ☐ No

Reasons for acceptance 1 _____

2 _____

3 _____

Reasons for refusal 1 _____

2 _____

3 _____

Action _____

_____

_____

_____

Signed _____ Position _____

Page 2 of 2

Chart 2.21: Sample Candidate Summaries

Name of child	Age	Dx	Medical information	Means of intake	Range of intake	Sensory	Self-feeding	Nutrition	OMD Yes/No	Aversion Yes/No	Carer concerns	Aversion signals
Ivan	4.0	ID	History reflux	PEG	Water	Will explore food & brush teeth	✗	↑	✗	✓ Selective	I'm focused on eating to a huge degree, 'fixated on feeding' child.	Throws food away, walks away
Gary	3.09	ID low tone	Fundoplication	Oral	Liquid Purée	Hyposensitive intraorally.	✗	→	✓	✓ Selective	Eats very little + slowly. Won't put hands to mouth, everything puréed	Turns away, Spillage, Vocalisations, Crying
Lorcan	4.11	?	Anti-epilepsy medicines	PEG	Nil orally	Rejects all stimuli – facial or oral	✗	↑	✗	✓ Total	Asks for things but doesn't eat, Licks only	Walks away, verbalises, Pretends to co-operate
Lucy	7.08	CP	Aspiration on thin liquids	PEG	Tastes only	Reacts to smells	✓	↑	✓ Swallow dysfunction	✓ Total	Worried about when she's older, want to get her eating before her friends start to notice	Spits out, Intraoral hold
Roisin	6.10	ASD		Oral	Liquids		✓	↑	↑	✓ Selective	Want to change her behaviour	Bites, spits, refuses spoon feeds
Stephen	5.01	CP	Gastro-oesophageal reflux (GOR) diagnosed	PEG + oral	Liquids	Hyposensitive	✗	↑	→	✓ Selective	To come off tube	Never cries for food, turns away, protrudes tongue, closes mouth

Key:

DX = Diagnosis
ASD = Autistic Spectrum Disorder
CP = Cerebral Palsy
ID = Intellectual disability

PEG = percutaneous endoscopic gastrostomy
Nutrition = weight. Arrows indicate above (↑), below (↓) or ideal weight (→).
OMD = information on oral motor function

Form 2.22: Sample Severity Ratings*

Rating	Food approach behaviour: sit with ease
1	Child will sit easily at the table
2	Occasionally child will be difficult to sit at the table or leave early
3	Frequently child will be difficult to sit at the table or will be in and out of the chair or leave early
4	Sometimes the child will sit, but it always takes a lot of effort Will be in and out of the chair all the time
5	Child will not go near a table or place where food also is present.

Rating	Food approach behaviour: time spent eating
1	Will eat like other children interspersed with chatting and fun
2	Takes a number of bites/drinks but not as much as carer would like
3	Will take bites or sips but carer can count on two hands the number of times this happens during a meal
4	Will eat or drink very rarely and it is effortful for child Spends more time thinking about eating than actually doing it
5	Will not eat or drink at all.

Rating	Eating & Drinking – range
1	No problems – child eats and drinks almost everything offered, similar to peers
2	Some little problems – occasionally refuses specific items of food or drink
3	Child gets by but carer has to plan every meal Refuses a lot of foods/drinks but not impossible to feed, or to take out
4	A lot of problems with food: although child will eat or drink something, it is limited Carer has considerable difficulty planning meals
5	Won't eat or drink at all Won't even touch or smell food Won't let anything near mouth or face like teeth brushing or face washing.

where 1 = normal/no aversion present in this area, and 5 = profound problems

Page 1 of 2

Form 2.22: *continued*

Rating	Sensory/tactile/activities of daily living responses
1	Just like other children with regard to teeth brushing, washing hands, face washing, hair brushing etc
2	Doesn't like activities like teeth brushing, face washing but does it daily
3	Doesn't like these activities Carer can do these activities some days but not every day by any means and it is an effort
4	Hates things like teeth brushing, face washing or getting hands dirty Occasionally, it can get done – once a week maybe but it is difficult
5	Won't let anyone touch face, mouth or hands.

Rating	Behavioural reactions
1	Doesn't react strongly to food or drink, similar to peers
2	Will comment or turn away occasionally but really child gets on with it Not too much fuss
3	Shows obvious dislike at every meal Despite this generally attempts eating
4	Will scream, cry, etc and will turn away physically from food or drink
5	Screams, runs away when food mentioned You couldn't put child in the same room as food He/she gets sick.

Rating	How much time/work carer spends/does to get child to eat – effects
1	No greater a time commitment than for other children
2	A little encouragement is needed Carer may have to work out something different for child sometimes
3	Needs a lot of thought Carer has to prepare especially for child, but it is achievable
4	Affects carer's life considerably Requires a lot of thought and effort but doesn't totally take over
5	A lot of time spent preparing, finding the right food or drink that child will eat, coercing them to actually eat Carer's day revolves around it.

* where 1 = normal/no aversion present in this area, and 5 = profound problems

Page 2 of 2

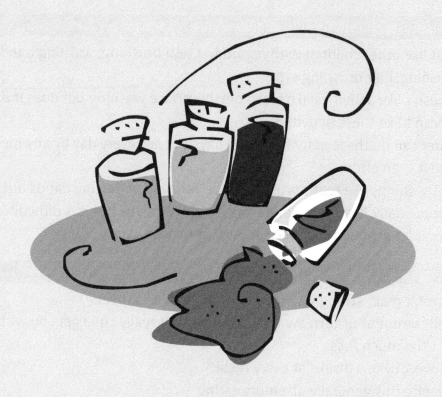

Chapter 3

STAGE 2

Food for Thought:
The carer programme

The Food for Thought carer programme is designed to meet the needs of carers of children with feeding aversion. It typically precedes direct intervention with the child, and focuses on developing the carer skills essential to the successful implementation of the programme for the child.

Training parents and carers is a core feature of the Fun with Food approach to oral feeding aversion for the following reasons. Training:

- promotes improved clinical effectiveness and appropriate management
- promotes safe practices and client care
- reduces anxiety experienced by carers and families
- facilitates development of understanding of therapy goals specifically, and eating & drinking & swallowing (EDS) generally
- improves interdisciplinary working
- improves communication within the team and between carers and team members
- allows for skill sharing between clinicians and carers, and between carers
- provides opportunities for peer support and establishment of rapport between clinicians and carers
- creates informed carers who become active participants in the intervention process
- motivates carers.

Fun with Food's carer training focus intends to provide a solid base to treatment which negates the impact of the factors such as those outlined by Colodny (2001), who found carers were 'non-compliant' with dysphagia recommendations, predominately due to:

- insufficient knowledge
- disagreement with the recommendations
- implementing recommendations was too much hassle and required different skills
- intervention guidelines were not concrete.

What is involved in training carers?

Carer education and development can be targeted, either in the form of a 'Carer Day' (without children) prior to the other elements of the course, or integrated into the Fun before Food (Chapter 4) and EDS (Chapter 5) elements of the programme. This will depend on the clinician's preference, and on resources available. However, by having a dedicated Carer Day prior to the child-based elements of the programme, carers will develop the knowledge and mindset that will help them approach therapy with more confidence and understanding, thereby facilitating intervention readiness.

Carer training involves a variety of approaches, including:

■ lectures
■ group brainstorming
■ problem-solving activities
■ experiential activities, including role-play.

Samples of these follow. The clinician should decide which activities are most appropriate for their service users.

Carer pack

The carer pack is essentially a folder containing course information and guidelines. Its purpose is threefold:

1 To prepare the carer for the programme by giving information on the different aspects of the programme.
2 To share information via guidelines, reports etc.
3 To provide a point for keeping all information gathered during the programme.

When is the carer pack given?

The carer pack is given to the carers on the morning of the Food for Thought carer programme. It can also be sent in advance. It includes the forms that can be found at the end of this chapter, namely:

■ Introduction Letter (Form 3.1)
■ Key-worker Handout (Form 3.2)
■ Aims Handout (Form 3.3)
■ Timetables for course elements (samples in Appendix 1)
■ Session handouts for programme activities (also included at the end of the chapter).

As more sessions are introduced, so too is material added to the pack.

Carer pack forms

Introduction Letter (Form 3.1)
Outlines the format of the course.

Key-worker Handout (Form 3.2)
The key-worker session occurs for the last half hour of every day of the Fun before Food and EDS programme days. It provides carers and a designated clinician with an opportunity to meet together at the end of each day to resolve any outstanding issues, facilitate carry-over of recommendations and strategies, and go over any areas which may need to be repeated for the benefit of either party. Carers are given a handout to explain how the system operates.

Aims Handout (Form 3.3)
This form outlines the aims of the programme and advises carers of the overall aim for each child, which is to increase oral nutritional intake. This aim will be long- or short-term depending on the individual. Specific aims are both long- and short-term, and will be discussed during the Food for Thought carer programme, on day 1 of the Eating & Drinking & Swallowing programme (through the orientation session) and again on the last day. Goal setting is a pivotal component of the programme, and carers benefit from having general aims clearly stated before they commence their own specific goal-setting practice.

Staff List Handout (Form 3.5)
It is important to ensure that carers and children know who staff are, and what their roles will be. This helps with familiarity and the directing of questions or issues to the right person. See Form 3.4 for a sample staff list.

What to Bring Handout (Form 3.6)
Carers are given details of what they need to bring with them to both the pre-feeding and EDS elements of the programme.

Carer Contact Numbers (Form 3.7)
Carers often find it useful to have each other's contact details. Provide carers with either a blank sheet they can fill in or, if you have received their permission, type their details onto the form and copy it to all carers.

Food for Thought carer programme sessions

There are three core areas which should be focused on during the carer programme, covering interaction, managing behaviour and nutrition, as these are seen as pivotal to the subsequent development of the child's EDS skills. In devising a timetable, the clinician should use a number of activity sessions from each of these areas. Additionally, it is possible to incorporate carer sessions into the EDS programme itself if it is felt carers need more of this type of approach. There are also other suggested activities to facilitate discussion, group bonding and carer development in other areas and these follow.

1 Orientation session (Form 3.8)

In essence, this session:

- Introduces staff and carers to each other
- Gives a general outline of the programme
- Goes through the initial carer handouts in the carer pack.

2 Nutrition session
Marie Kennedy

The aim of this session is to provide a basic overview of nutrition to facilitate the carer's understanding of the nutritional requirements for their children. Topics in this section should be relevant to both developing a general understanding of nutrition and highlighting any areas relevant to the group as a whole or individuals within the group.

Activity suggestions

Nutritional overview
Using charts and diagrams explain:

- The use of weight and height charts and how ideal body weight is achieved
- The function and source of energy, protein, fat, vitamins and minerals
- Nutritional deficiencies such as anaemia, rickets.

Issues in nutrition and the disabled child

Discuss and brainstorm, for example:

- Oral motor dysfunction and its relation to nutritional intake
- Failure to thrive and grow
- Constipation.

Fluid intake

Discuss:

- Role of fluids
- Balance between solid and fluid intake and potential to overfill with fluids in attempts to improve oral intake
- Fluids and appetite suppression
- Necessity for children to receive sufficient fluids daily
- Signs of dehydration (see handout, Form 3.9).

Use of supplements

- Define 'What are supplements?' The clinician can exhibit various brands
- Discuss when supplements should be recommended
- Discuss supplements and oral intake.

Tube feeding

- Why is tube feeding used? Carers who have children who are tube feeding can demonstrate their knowledge by answering this and presenting their child's history to the group. This can help facilitate discussion and group bonding.
- Is tube feeding permanent?
- Balancing tube and oral feeding generally, and in the context of the Fun with Food programme's focus on developing oral eating skills and improving intake.

Discuss possible weight loss

- Discuss the nutritional stability of all children prior to the programme and the constant weight monitoring by the dietitian within the programme which facilitates confidence in pursuing EDS goals.
- Discuss the possibility of weight loss in the context working on EDs aversion. Remind carers of the daily monitoring by the programme's dietitian. Inform carers that the dietitian sees the carers and children first thing every morning of the EDS element of the programme to monitor the children's weight, fluid and solid intake and tube-feeding regime.

3 Interaction

Feeding is one of the most natural experiences between carer and child, and provides a unique opportunity for bonding and social experiences. When feeding goes wrong, the interaction between the individual being fed, and the carer who feeds, may suffer. Carers can over- or under-compensate, can read the child's signals inappropriately, and the boundaries between appropriate and inappropriate signals and responses can become confused. This is not surprising in the context of the carer's desire to ensure adequate nutritional intake and the development of oral feeding.

This section of the carer programme plans to develop awareness of the carer's interaction styles and the child's communication signals, and how these individually and combined may be influencing the outcome and development of oral eating skills. Videotaping is used to facilitate skill development. The value of videotaping should not be under-rated in facilitating the intervention process, particularly as:

- It concentrates the mind and facilitates the memory through audio and visual feedback
- It can provide numerous examples. There are opportunities for repetition
- It is concrete – carers can relate to it
- Carers can see children similar to their own. It reduces isolation and self-blame thoughts
- It is a system of record keeping – can chart progress
- It is child-specific rather than generalisation-based
- Seeing is believing.

Activity suggestions

A number of activity suggestions are listed here, and the clinician can choose which they will utilise. However, it is suggested that the last, which focuses on the main principles of good interaction, always be included.

Why does EDS interaction go wrong?

Brainstorm how and why EDS interaction can go wrong, resultant feelings and pressures to feed orally.

What I do as a carer and what my child does during EDS that helps or hinders my child's eating

Get carers to provide a written account (and present it to the group), or brainstorm what their child does, and what they do as a carer, that both negatively and positively influences EDS interactions.

Analyse samples of EDS interactions

Use videotape examples of EDS interactions from other aversive feeders to get carers to take an objective view of 'good' and 'poor' carer–child EDS interactions. Use open questions such as 'What do you think is positive about this interaction?' and 'What do you think this carer could change?'

Rate examples of EDS interactions

Carers rate videotape examples of EDS interactions using the Interaction Rating Form (Form 3.10), which can be used to guide the process. This facilitates the development of carer observation and analytic skills. Identify additional behaviours to enter on the form based on the videos selected.

Individual interaction analysis

Use videos taken on the Assessment Day to commence individual interaction analysis. This should be done in the carer group rather than individually. (Form 3.12 provides a template for summarising Assessment Day interactions.) This fosters a peer support approach as well as reducing self-blame, which can hinder progress. Carers are encouraged to:

- Provide a commentary on their own video – it is wise to pre-select about one to three minutes of the tape which includes both positive and non-positive interactions.
- Identify one item they would change from their own video, while other carers watching are asked to choose one positive carer interaction or behaviour.
- Review the tape and ask carers to comment on the child's communication signals or behaviours, both verbal and non-verbal (eg throwing food, leaving table, using questions to distract) using the Child Communication Signals Form (Form 3.11). The carer should provide feedback to the group and finish with identification of the good points each child brings to the EDS situation.

Each carer, with the help of the clinician, should select for practice in the intervening time between the carer programme and EDS programme, a single carer behaviour to change. Alternatively or in addition (depending on the individual carers and group), each carer should select a single child communication signal for which to watch out and adapt their reaction.

Discuss interaction styles

Discuss different carer interaction styles. Get carers to describe their style of interaction using between one and three labels. This will help them frame more clearly how they interact with their child. Terms previously encountered include 'mothering', 'teacher', 'drill sergeant'. Discuss the pros and cons of each of these styles.

Role-play positive and negative interaction styles when pretend-feeding.

Examples are given in Table 15.

It can be useful to type up a list of sample behaviours and place individual ones in an envelope, give the envelope to the carer who will role-play the behaviour, and encourage the other carers to identify what behaviour was being role-played. Carers should alternate so they have an opportunity to be both carer and child in role-play scenarios, and after each role-play they should discuss how it felt to be the child and carer in turn.

Main interaction principles

Discuss the main interaction principles (see Form 3.13) for EDS management during the programme as identified in the handout at the end of the chapter. Based on the make-up of the carer group attending the course, the clinician may want to include other simple rules which target specific individual behaviours.

4 Managing behaviour

Facilitate the carer and their child to move forward by the provision of a supportive and logical environment. This can be achieved through discussion of the points outlined below. A dedicated session on behaviour management led by a psychologist may also benefit carers.

- **Reframe the carer's construction of behaviours**, for example as 'boldness'. Many behaviours around mealtime can be construed as a child being bold. While the child may have behavioural/management problems, these often reflect fear of eating and coping or avoidance issues. Many children express real fear around food, for example through statements such as 'You're trying to poison me'. Ask carers to identify what emotions their children are really feeling. Eating is not a pleasant experience for many children with feeding aversion.
- **Boundaries**. Children respond well to boundaries. They require these to understand what is acceptable and what is not acceptable, and to be able therefore to move forward. Boundaries facilitate development of trust.

Table 15: Samples of interaction behaviours

Constructive
▪ Encouraging the child verbally and non-verbally
▪ Giving the child space and time to eat
▪ You decide! The rest of the group guess what it is you do to help the child
▪ Smiling
▪ Modelling eating
▪ Positive facial expression
▪ Consistency between carers

Non-constructive
▪ Constantly urging to eat. Trying to get the child to eat more and quicker, offer opinions on the food, eg 'Try it', 'Come on', 'Have some more', 'Bite it', 'Mmm, it's lovely', ' It's nice'
▪ Reminding the child that if he doesn't eat he won't grow to be big and strong
▪ Carer standing while feeding the child – always looking down on the child
▪ Talking incessantly – topic doesn't matter
▪ Not talking at all – giving no feedback to the child
▪ Goals are too big – unwieldy, eg telling the child to eat two bowls of pasta, three pieces of bread etc
▪ Using lots of questions – eg 'Will you eat this for your mother, please'
▪ Pretending to force feed
▪ Keep changing the goals – every time the child does what is asked, make a new goal
▪ Making threats
▪ Pleading with the child
▪ Getting angry with the child
▪ Telling the child that the other carer won't be happy if he doesn't eat
▪ Telling the child that he won't go to … (somewhere nice) etc, if he doesn't eat

- **Ask 'Who is the boss?'** Encourage carers to review their interactions with their children around EDS and answer the above question. Typically, role reversal has occurred and children are managing to control the behaviour of the carers. Motivate the carers to take control again.
- **Think small.** Don't let the EDS problem be so big in carers' minds that it becomes unmanageable. Facilitate them to deal with it by thinking in terms of small, progressive steps, and through setting clear goals. See goal-setting discussion below.
- **Model social eating** by encouraging carers and child to eat together, and make this a positive time for carer and children.

- **Use praise for achieving goals**. Improve the EDS environment. Carers should not overdo praise but provide it only for achieving goals they have set. Praise should be immediate and contingent on achieving goals.
- **Do not discuss EDS issues and the child's performance in front of the child**, either during or outside of the eating context. Children can pick up on a carer's worries from overhearing discussions. Only discuss concerns when the child is well out of earshot. If the child wants to get into a discussion with the carer about EDS issues, including goals, the carer should not oblige him. The carer should create the expectation that goals will be met.
- **Consistency between carers is the key**. It is important for carers to agree on goals and management prior to EDS activities so that mixed messages are not given. More failures can result from the inability of carers to be consistent than from any other area.
- **Use reinforcement**. What type is up to the carer and based on their knowledge of the child, but this should be decided before the EDS element of the programme. Reinforcement should be consequent on achieving the set goal, and immediate. Carers should not resort to arguments such as 'No you didn't do what I wanted so I am not going to give you ...' If a goal is not achieved, carers should simply not supply the reinforcement/reward. When a child achieves the set goal, the carer should frame the child's achievement, no matter how small, positively. Reinforcement should always be individualised and in proportion to the child's achievement. Use a reinforcement chart – accumulative – if appropriate. Do not choose food as reinforcement. Extinguish the reward frequency as the child progresses.
- **Develop goal-setting skills**. See Form 3.20 and the EDS programme, Chapter 5.

5 Worst-case scenario

This brainstorm session can often be best used in the middle of the EDS component of the programme as carers confront the realities of changing their behaviour and attitudes, and as the group bond develops.

Carers describe what, in their opinion, is the worst that can happen with regard to EDS. The origin of this discussion comes from fear. Some carers may be reluctant to embrace the EDS programme because they fear certain events – worst-case scenarios, such as tantrums in a restaurant, choking and so on.

In this discussion carers are given a few minutes to define what exactly for them is the worst-case scenario with regard to their child's eating and drinking. This is a situation that has probably already happened, and that carers found either distressing or were unable to cope with at that time. Carers:

- identify their worst case scenario
- inform the group
- pair off and 'counsel' each other in turn.

It is surprising, once carers are put in positions to help others, how successful this can be. Clinicians rarely need to provide any answers – the carers find answers for each other, and often come up with great solutions, or just a listening ear. When the carers have finished this exercise, each carer feeds back their initial scenario, their current thoughts on it, and any solutions or resolutions suggested or identified.

6 Mealtime structure

This session is utilised to develop routine and structure around mealtimes, to facilitate development of boundaries. Carers should:

- Outline their own and child's routines with times on a flip chart.
- Draw a table with family's places, in which rooms etc.
- Explain their mealtime routines to other carers.
- Comment on their own and each other's routines both positively and with suggestions for change. Discuss the message the child receives with elements from each carer's routine.
- Discuss lifestyles, various individual and family needs, and how this impacts on mealtime structure.
- Discuss best practice and why routines are important from both nutritional and child comprehension points of view.
- 'Draw' their goals for best practice in this area.

7 Food memories

The aim of this session is not to analyse in detail carers' responses to food in detail. It is more a facilitative exercise to develop carer analysis about their approach to food, which may be affecting their ability to help their child. For example, at this stage some carers are so concerned about nutritional intake that they find it difficult to take risks with setting goals. Whether this is a result of the child's EDS difficulties or whether it existed prior to them is not the issue here; what the clinician is aspiring to, is encouraging self-analysis to facilitate progress. Any major issues that are felt to verge on carer eating disorder should be referred on to the relevant professional with carer approval. The clinician may want to use mnemonics such as old cartons of food or photos of old fashioned shops. Start the discussion off generally, then move towards scripting memories.

Carers should:

■ Write down two food memories – one really positive, one really negative. How did these events influence them?
■ Tell other carers about their family's approach and attitude to food. How did this influence them?

8 Carer therapy tips – what works and what doesn't?

This brainstorm session may be best used towards the end of the EDS programme. Carers can teach and support each other through this activity.

Advise carers to:

■ Share with the group any tips or strategies they have found useful that may help others. For example, carers have previously identified their tips as:
  – Persistence
  – Co-operative working
  – Being able to call the dietitian
  – Not giving up
  – Keeping a blank facial expression
  – Modelling
  – Understanding where the children are coming from (through doing the experiential eating exercise)
  – Placing food for all the family in the middle of the table on a plate rather than placing the child's food on the child's plate.
■ Tell other carers one thing they have found that definitely does not work.

9 The most difficult thing about EDS problems

This session gives carers an opportunity to discuss how hard it can be to have a child with an EDS problems, and to provide peer support. The discussion can be opened up by provision of examples given by carers previously such as:

- It's hard to take away our dependence on formula and trust that we will be able to get him to eat 'normal' foods
- It is really hard to watch other kids eat normally
- If I can't feed my kid, which is his most basic of needs, and the thing all other parents can do, then I must be a bad mother.

10 Expectations

It is important to hold a discussion, however brief, on carer expectations. There can be an expectation by the carers that the programme will provide a miraculous solution to their children's EDS problems, such that they will finish the programme experiencing no further difficulties. To this end it is important to:

- Elicit carer expectations
- Discuss carer roles – active partners in process
- Reinforce the need for a step-by-step approach
- Discuss how the process of change can be slow and sometimes frustrating. Use analogies such as adults who try to lose weight.

11 Experiential eating

This session aims to provide the carer with perspective on a child's reactions to food he does not like, put the child's responses into perspective, and increase the carer's understanding of their child's mealtime experience.

- Provide a brief overview of the theory behind sensory processing problems to enable carers to better understand the way in which their child receives information from the environment and the way in which he responds to this information.
- Get carers to discuss their biggest fear, for example fear of heights, or discuss reality TV shows where people have to eat 'obnoxious' items. Ask carers to put themselves into this situation and equate it to the fear their child feels on being asked to take a new food.
- Undertake role-play/participation exercises such as:
  (a) Work with spouse or other carer in group. Carer should be fed by other carer, preferably blindfolded. The tastes used in this can be common such as yoghurts and mashed potatoes but the person being fed should not know what it is. Get carers to discuss the experience afterwards. How did it feel to have so little control? Not knowing what the taste was going to be?

(b) Based on the Tastes & Textures Questionnaire previously filled out, carers will have identified their least favourite foods. The clinician should have purchased these in preparation for this session. These can vary significantly, from what some people would consider 'normal' foods such as cheese to less normal foods such as snails and oysters. The clinician will often have had to do a little shopping around for this session – but it is worth the effort for the right results. Carers should have to eat their hated foods. Provide tissues or utensils for spitting out! Discuss how difficult it is to eat something you don't like. Invite carers to describe their physical and emotional reaction to the disliked foods.

12 Sensory diet
Jeni Malone

The aim of this session is to facilitate a greater understanding of sensory processing and of the difficulties that can be experienced by children, and thus enable carers to better understand some of their child's behaviour and discover how to manage this more successfully through the use of appropriate activities at intervals throughout the day. The clinician will provide information and facilitate a discussion on sensory processing problems and sensory diet.

Each carer should have the opportunity to work with the clinician to identify activities appropriate for their child, and set up a sensory diet which can be integrated into their home/family life (this can happen at a later stage if full sensory assessment has not been completed and discussed with the carers). Some of the points covered in this session are listed in Table 16.

A blank Sensory Diet Sheet (Form 3.15) is given to carers along with a Sample Sensory Diet Sheet (Form 3.14). This will provide them with a clearer idea of how the different types of sensory activities can be used. Activity ideas should also be discussed, identifying those that might help alert/arouse a child's activity level and those that might help to calm/organise a child. Carers can identify specific times of the day or specific daily tasks that are most challenging for their child and can incorporate activities as required, for example deep pressure activities before teeth-brushing and feeding to calm/prepare the child.

Sensory activity suggestions and examples are listed in Table 17 on page 114.

For other activity ideas refer to Yack et al (1998) and Stock Kranowitz (2003).

Table 16: Sample sensory Questions & Answers

Question	Answer
What is sensory processing?	Our link with the external environment from our internal environment.
What is sensory information?	It is what we feel, see and hear.
What are our sensory systems?	Visual, auditory, olfactory, gustatory, somatosensory, vestibular, proprioceptive. The tactile, vestibular and proprioceptive systems are fundamental and closely connected. They develop in utero and work together in an integrated and automatic way. We gather the information into our nervous system, which interprets the information and responds with a behaviour.
What is a difficulty with sensory processing?	In order to react to different situations we have to interpret the information appropriately. In order to interpret the information appropriately we have to gather it accurately. A difficulty with sensory processing does not mean that the brain is damaged, but that the information from the senses is not flowing and integrating efficiently.
What is the aim of intervention?	Intervention is a process of learning to enable the child to process information in a more effective way. Activities are designed to gradually increase the demand on the child to make an organised response and perform tasks with greater skill (based on Bundy et al, 1991).
What is a sensory diet?	A planned and scheduled activity programme designed to meet a child's specific sensory needs. The 'main course' includes movement, deep touch pressure and heavy work. 'Snacks' include other types of activities involving the mouth and auditory, visual and smell experiences.
What is the purpose of a sensory diet?	To provide the combination of sensory input which is just right to achieve and maintain optimal levels of arousal and performance in the neurological system. To reduce protective or sensory defensiveness that can negatively affect social contact, interaction and learning (Wilbarger, 1995; Wilbarger & Wilbarger, 2001).
What is the sensory profile and how is it relevant?	The 'sensory profile' is a caregiver questionnaire which allows us to look at a child's responses to sensory input, to see if these are indicative of a sensory processing difficulty, and to aid in development of intervention planning (Dunn, 1999a – see the section on sensory processing assessment).

Table 17: Sensory activity suggestions and examples

Sensory-based activities	Activities
Proprioceptive	Heavy marching
	Chair/wall push-ups
	Body squeezes
	Wheelbarrow walks
	Foot-to-foot cycling
	Heavy jobs eg carrying books, moving furniture, cleaning the blackboard
	Crash pad
	Tug of war
	Theraband™ (available from physiotherapy suppliers)
	Play wrestling
Tactile	Feely boxes with variety of toys to explore, eg balls, brushes, feathers
	Hidden objects in sand, eg buttons, beads, blocks, small toys (cars, animals)
	Hidden objects in putty
	Variety of tactile art media, eg paint with sponges, fingers
	Collage work with variety of paper, card, material
	Hand massage
	Play with shaving foam
	Tactile road, ie variety of materials to walk on with hands or feet
	Dress-up games
	Hot dog roll, ie rolling child up in blanket
Vestibular	Sitting or prone on therapy ball – singing activities while bouncing to the beat, playing throw and catch with balls, beanbags
	Jumping on trampoline
	Slides/swings/see-saw
	Rocking chair
	Play wrestling
	Wheelbarrows
	Running/jumping/spinning

continued →

Table 17: *continued*

Sensory-based activities	Activities
Auditory	Tapping beats of tunes
	Matching sounds
	Co-ordinating words of songs with actions
	The clinician may need to filter out extraneous auditory information, eg if the child has auditory defensiveness, he may need a quiet environment to facilitate participation in other activities
Gustatory/olfactory	Smell and tell games
	Scented cards
	Taste and tell
	Gel pens

13 Normal EDS development

Carers can be given handouts or provided with references for detailed information on normal EDS development (eg Evans Morris & Dunn Klein 1987, Winstock 1994, McCurtin 1997). In addition, there are some videos (eg Normal Oral Motor & Swallowing Development: Birth to 36 months; Channel 4's 'Baby it's You' and 'Life Before Birth') that provide useful edited representations of normal EDS development. Samples of development in various different EDS areas are included at the end of the chapter (Forms 3.16–3.19), and can form the bases of discussions. The questions and answers outlined in Table 18 should also help give structure to this session.

Other areas of consideration might include:

1 The impact of cognitive development.
2 The eating and social environments of the child.
3 The cultural environment. Winstock (1994) comments on certain foods prohibited in some cultures, later weaning practices, table seating arrangements, whether utensils or fingers are used, etc.
4 Family preferences.
5 Individual likes and dislikes and individual variation.
6 Transitions. Some cultures do not dwell on transitional feeding, some do.
7 The 'critical period'. For the first three years, humans are programmed for development of EDS and speech skills. It is easier to develop critical skills during this time than after (Chapman Bahr, 2001).

Table 18: Normal EDS development Questions & Answers

Question	Sample answer
Why discuss normal development?	Frame of reference against which we measure current, normal and abnormal skills Building blocks for creating treatment programmes (Evans Morris & Dunn Klein, 1987) Complex process which is influenced by multiple factors Framework for rational conceptualisation, evaluation and management (Stevenson & Allaire, 1996).
What disrupts normal development?	Examples: Prematurity – The immature central nervous system may be overly sensitive to a multitude of stimuli Chronic illness – The child's resources are harnessed towards survival Delayed introduction to normal development with regard to liquids and solids, eg naso-gastric feeding, can bypass normal development Unpleasant oral tactile experiences, eg intubation (Wolf & Glass 1992) Impaired feeding experiences Conditions such as cerebral palsy, Down syndrome **Activity suggestion** Brainstorm – What do you think disrupted your child's EDS development? Carers should provide feedback to group and discuss.
What is normal EDS development dependent on?	Anatomical integrity Experiential learning is crucial. Eating and swallowing are such natural, subconscious acts that many adults forget that eating is a learned skill – most of feeding is a learned behaviour (Stevenson & Allaire, 1996) There is an orderly sequence of acquisition of skills It parallels psychological, cognitive and social/emotional milestones. Especially parallels gross and fine motor development (Walter, 1994).

continued ➜

Table 18: *continued*

Question	Sample answer
What are reflexes?	Two categories: *Adaptive*. Adaptive assists in feeding-functional reflex, eg sucking, rooting *Protective*. Protects the airway/digestive tract against foreign matter. Expels foreign matter, eg cough, gag Feeding reflexes present at birth evolve with modification over time into adult-like patterns by approximately three years of age. The presence of reflexes beyond the age at which they typically disappear can signal neurological impairment (McKeever Murphy & Caretto, 1997), and behavioural/aversive issues **Activity suggestion** In aversive children, you will sometimes see overdeveloped use of the cough and gag reflexes. Carers should discuss the differences between the cough and gag reflexes and brainstorm how they would know if one of these reflexes was being used behaviourally or as the result of safety issues, eg aspiration.

8 Reversion. The acquisition of new skills can cause reversion to earlier patterns of oral motor skill; for example introduction of a purée/cracker. Experience is required to learn to manipulate new food textures in different ways from previous textures, and reversion happens as 'a more difficult component of movement is perfected' (Stephenson & Allaire, 1996). Some of the previously learned postural control and stability is forfeited (Evans Morris & Dunn Klein, 1987*)*.

9 Implications of diagnosis on EDS skills development. For example, natural progression does not happen in children with cerebral palsy or other neurological disorders.

14 Goal setting

Goal setting is the most important skill carers will learn. If they can manage to learn to goal set appropriately, relative to their child's needs, they can ensure success for their child and themselves. The aim of this skill is to facilitate carers to learn to grade their expectations of their child and make the 'big', apparently overwhelming, EDS problem workable, to focus on small achievable areas which are remediable and achievable. Carers are encouraged to think in terms of small steps. In this session the principles of goal setting are discussed using Form 3.20 at the end of the chapter. The principles should always be discussed by giving examples. Specific goal-setting training should take place in the Eating & Drinking & Swallowing programme for each EDS activity.

15 Formalising aims

At the end of the Food for Thought carer programme, or prior to the Eating & Drinking & Swallowing programme, carers are asked to use Form 3.21 to define what exactly they require from the course. These aims can be as broad or as narrow as they like. Staff will have made their own goals after the Assessment Day for each child and these should be typed up immediately after completion, using Form 3.22, and given to carers at this time, as well as copied to the child's file. This facilitates discussion of carer and clinician aims for the child, serves to facilitate communication, co-operation, goal-setting skills and so on. Often, this process helps carers understand their that aims may be too ambitious for their child. These aims are returned to at the end of the EDS part of the programme and again on More Food Review Days, to help refocus both staff and carers, and reframe aims if necessary.

Examples of a team's goals for a child are to:

- Increase range of tastes beyond sweet foods
- Increase range of consistencies taken within oral motor abilities
- Increase range of temperature taken
- Analyse oral motor function
- Reduce stress of feeding
- Reduce fluid intake where it is preventing intake of solids
- Remove tube feeding entirely
- Develop self-feeding.

16 Feedback on Food for Thought carer programme

Carers are asked to rate the carer programme sessions using Form 3.23. Feedback received will facilitate development of both current and future programmes.

Chapter 3 Photocopiable master forms and sample forms

Carer programme sessions

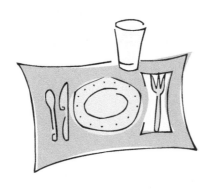

Form 3.1: Introduction Letter

Dear Carer

Welcome!

As you know the Fun with Food programme is split into five main sections:

1 The Assessment Day, which you have already completed.

2 The Food For Thought carer programme – a dedicated carer (no children) day for training and talking.

3 The pre-feeding programme Fun before Food – for you and your child to work on skills that support EDS development. There is no focus on actual eating during this element of the course.

4 The Eating & Drinking & Swallowing programme. This section of the course focuses on actual opportunities to work on EDS skills. There will be four to five opportunities each day for you and your child to work on eating skills.

5 More Food Review Days. These are held at timed intervals to facilitate carry-over, address any outstanding issues, monitor progress and continue EDS work.

Participation

All elements of the programme are mandatory unless otherwise agreed in advance with the course co-ordinator.

Information

You will be provided with more information about each element as the programme proceeds.

Partnership

Our philosophy is that this programme works best if clinicians and carers work closely in partnership with each other – as a team. Clinicians are there to empower and guide carers. You are encouraged to take an active part in your child's skill development. We look forward to working with you.

Page 1 of 2

Form 3.1: *continued*

Programme dates

These are the dates of the Fun with Food programme:

Programme component	Date
Assessment Day	
Food for Thought carer programme	
Fun before Food (pre-feeding programme)	
Eating & Drinking & Swallowing programme	
More Food Review Day 1 (1 month)	
Even More Food Review Day 2 (3 months)	
Review Day 3 (6 months)	
Review Day 4 (1 year)	

These dates are now firmly set. If you cannot make any of these dates, please let the course co-ordinator know as soon as possible.

_____ (Course co-ordinator)

Signed

Form 3.2: Key-worker Handout

Your key-worker is allocated when you are offered a place on the programme and is:

Name _____ **Telephone** _____

Aim

The key-worker session occurs for the last half hour of every day of the Fun before Food and EDS days. It provides you and a designated clinician with an opportunity to meet together at the end of each day to resolve any outstanding issues, facilitate carry-over of recommendations and strategies, and go over any areas that may need to be repeated for the benefit of either party.

While staff are more than happy to answer specific questions during sessions or activities during the day, any detailed queries you may have or points that need clarification should be kept until your key-worker session, when you will have a dedicated half hour with your allocated key-worker. Please use this time as effectively as possible.

Your key-worker's role is to facilitate your child's progress and co-ordinate with other staff members on your behalf if required.

Name of course co-ordinator _____

Telephone _____

The course co-ordinator is also more than happy to meet with you if requested.

Form 3.3: Aims Handout

The overall aim for each child is to increase oral nutritional intake. This aim will be long- or short-term depending on the individual.

Specific aims are both long- and short-term and will be discussed during the Food for Thought carer programme or on day one of the Eating & Drinking & Swallowing programme (through the orientation session) and on the last day. A discussion of aims is also bound to crop up during key-worker sessions.

Overall Eating & Drinking & Swallowing aims
- Decrease dependency on tube feeding (where present) for nutritional purposes
- Increase oral intake
- Extend range of tastes and textures taken orally.

General aims
- Provide support and peer support for carers
- Build up confidence around feeding
- Increase pleasure factor of feeding.

Programme goals
- The Fun with Food programme has three overriding elements:

Support
- To give carers opportunities to share ideas, issues and concerns with other carers who are in similar situations.

Education
- To help carers gain a broader understanding of how children develop eating & drinking skills and provide strategies to help skills develop.

Application
- To provide opportunities for carers to practise strategies under guidance
- To give opportunities to children to develop pre-feeding skills
- To support the development of eating & drinking skills through a structured immersion approach in a peer environment.

Form 3.4: Sample Staff List

Name	Role	Programme element	Lead
	Course co-ordinator	Eating activities Food for Thought Carer Day	Eating & Drinking & Swallowing programme Lectures
	Dietitian	Eating & Drinking & Swallowing programme Fun before Food	Weigh-ins Growing Big & Strong
	Occupational therapist	Fun before Food	Sensory sessions
	Speech & language therapist	Fun before Food	Food Play Oral Motor Skills
	Therapy assistant	Fun before Food Eating & Drinking & Swallowing programme	Homework time Child minding
	Counsellor	Eating & Drinking & Swallowing programme	Carer support groups

Form 3.5: Staff List Handout

For your information, this is a list of clinicians who will be working with you on the Fun with Food programme.

Name	Role	Programme element	Lead

Form 3.6: What to Bring Handout

In order to make your child's and your own experience as rewarding as possible please make sure you bring:

Fun before Food

Second set of clothes (for both of you!)

Aprons

Any favoured food/drinks for lunch and break times

Utensils

Favourite child activities, eg toys

Appropriate seating equipment

Eating & Drinking & Swallowing

Second set of clothes (for both of you!)

Aprons

Any favoured food/drinks for eating and drinking activities

Utensils

Favourite child activities, eg toys

Appropriate seating equipment

You are also advised to wear old clothes for the duration of the programme.

Please also advise the course co-ordinator of any allergies or suspected allergies you or your child may have.

Form 3.7: Carer Contact Numbers

Carer/s name/s	Child's name	Home tel no.	Mobile no.

Form 3.8: Orientation Letter

Introduction
- Staff & staff roles
- Carers & carer roles.

Timetable
- Introduce timetable
- Agree more Food Review dates.

Housekeeping
- Kitchen access
- General housekeeping.

Main principles
- Focus on pre-eating and drinking skills to support the development of EDS skills and target any specific issues that may arise which would hinder the development of those skills
- Peer-group support for carers and children
- Kick-start EDS skills
- Interdisciplinary approach
- Active carer participation and follow-through.

Objectives
Clinicians
- To work collaboratively with each other and carers to develop oral eating, drinking and swallowing skills in children with EDS difficulties
- To provide strategies and support to carers.

Form 3.8: *continued*

Carers
- To provide peer and professional support, education, facilitate application of strategies to develop oral feeding
- To meet carer goals for improvements to oral feeding.

Child
- To develop oral feeding skills relative to each child's pre-course performance in this area.

Assessment Day
- Analysis of the oral and non-oral eating habits of each child; nutritional and medical status
- Analysis of carer attitudes and interaction styles
- Determine whether each child meets the criteria for selection to the programme.

Food for Thought carer programme
- To provide an opportunity for carers to discuss issues without children present
- To provide education
- To introduce carers to peers and staff
- To respond to initial concerns
- To define goals.

Fun before Food programme
- To develop pre-feeding skills which will support the development of EDS skills
- To provide a lead-in for carers and children to EDS activities
- To familiarise children with oral and eating related issues and activities
- To develop a mindset in children that constructs oral and feeding activities positively.

Form 3.8: *continued*

Eating & Drinking & Swallowing programme

- To provide an interdisciplinary intensive course for aversive oral eaters and their carers to facilitate development of oral intake
- To develop oral eating habits in children
- To provide strategies for development of oral eating
- To facilitate development of carer attitudes to their child's oral eating
- To provide peer support for children and peer and professional support for carers
- To educate carers
- To facilitate carry-over of development into 'normal' environments.

More Food Review Days

- To assess progress
- To provide further strategies for continued development of oral eating skills in children
- To provide support to carers to continue development of oral eating skills without professional support
- To further facilitate continuation of carry-over of oral eating behaviours into home environments.

Form 3.9: Signs of Dehydration Handout

Appropriate fluid intake is essential for your child for many reasons, and you may find balancing this with your child's developing eating skills difficult. Please discuss any concerns you may have with the programme's dietitian and take care to monitor for the following signs of dehydration.

IN PARTICULAR WATCH OUT FOR

Poor urinary output

Constipation

Headaches

Confusion

Lethargy

Urinary tract infections

Form 3.10: Interaction Rating Form

Watch the video and rate the carer you observe for the following interactions.

Did the carer...	Never	Sometimes	Always
State what they expect child to do			
Use praise appropriately			
Use questions			
Emanate authority			
Set expectations			
Give undue attention			
Appear to be in control			
Plead			
Bribe, barter or negotiate			
Model 'good' eating and drinking skills			
Appear calm			
Be social – chatty and friendly			
Talk only or mostly about food			
Encourage the child			

Form 3.11: Child Communication Signals Form

Name of child _____ Date _____

Name of carer filling in the form _____

Describe what the child did to communicate	Describe what the carer did in response

Form 3.12: Summary of Assessment Day Interactions

Name of carer _____   Date _____

Child's name	Constructive interaction skills	Non-constructive interaction skills

Signed _____

Position _____

Form 3.13: Main Interaction Principles Handout

Remove all overt emotions from the process – detach yourself while interacting – be neutral.

Remove attention – negative (even if child fails) and positive – from the EDS process except to reward the child for achieving goals.

Be language-specific – identify and use keywords relevant to the goal – this means no negotiating.

Do not use questions. They open up the possibility of refusal.

Focus only on the goals and do not be distracted from them. State and repeat the goal as necessary.

Model good behaviour.

Form 3.14: Sample Sensory Diet Sheet

Name of child _____ Date _____

Proprioceptive-based activities

1 For example for wake-up routine: heavy marching, chair/wall push-ups, body squeezes, wheelbarrow walk, crab walk

2 For example for bedtime routine: deep pressure/hugs, rolling up tight in blanket

3 Pushing/lifting heavy objects such as toys, books, moving kitchen chair, setting table for dinner, sweeping

4 Rough-housing, play wrestling, foot-to-foot cycling, jumping on a small trampoline.

Vestibular-based activities

1 For example for wake-up routine: sitting on a ball/rocking chair

2 For example for bedtime routine: slow rocking

3 Slides, swings, monkey bars, sitting on a ball/peanut roll.

Tactile activities

1 Feely boxes, hidden objects in sand box, pasta, rice

2 Dough, putty, variety of tactile art material, paints (finger, sponges)

3 Variety of balls, soft toys, brushes.

Remember
Do not force your child to do more than they are ready to do.
Identify key times in your child's day when activities are needed/appropriate.

Form 3.14: *continued*

Time	Key events in day	Sensory diet activities
	Wake-up	Wake-up routine
	Teeth brushing	Incorporate deep-pressure activities to body
	Prior to breakfast	Biting hard & releasing
	Lunch	Blowing bubbles
	Play	Incorporating rough-housing and other activity ideas
	Dinner	Sucking in cheeks
	Bathing	Heavy rubdown before/after bath, lotion applied firmly
	Hair care	Deep pressure to torso, limbs, scalp Wear heavy blanket during haircut
	Bedtime	Bedtime routine

Page 2 of 2

Form 3.15: Sensory Diet Sheet

Name of child _____   Date _____

Proprioceptive-based activities

1 _____
_____

2 _____
_____

3 _____
_____

Vestibular-based activities

1 _____
_____

2 _____
_____

3 _____
_____

Tactile activities

1 _____
_____

2 _____
_____

3 _____
_____

Remember
Do not force your child to do more than they are ready to do.
Identify key times in your child's day when activities are needed/appropriate.

Page 1 of 2

Form 3.15: *continued*

Time	Key events in day	Sensory diet activities
	Wake-up	Wake-up routine
	Breakfast	
	Lunch	
	Dinner	
	Bedtime	Bedtime routine

Page 2 of 2

Form 3.16: Examples of EDS Development by Structure

THE LIPS

Age	Note	Reference
6 months	Lower lip can protrude independently under a utensil to provide stability	Alexander (1987)
9 months	Upper lip actively removes food from spoon	Winstock (1994)
12–18 months	Make a seal when drinking	Winstock (1994)
By 18 months	Chew with lips closed – with intermittent mouth opening except during swallowing	Winstock (1994)
To 24 months	Food and saliva loss due to incomplete lip closure	Winstock (1994)
By 36 months	Lip seal complete in feeding	Winstock (1994)

THE TONGUE

Age	Note	Reference
Up to 6 months	Habitual thrusting pattern	McCurtin (1997)
At 6 months	In chewing, tongue moves up and down in a munching pattern	Evans Morris & Dunn Klein (1987)
7 months	In chewing, tongue moves up and down in a munching pattern	Evans Morris & Dunn Klein (1987)
From 12 months	Transfer centre to side initially with a pause in transfer	Winstock (1994)
At 12 months	Tongue may protrude slightly under cup to provide stability	
12–18 months	Rotary tongue movement	Winstock (1994)
24 months	Can transfer side to side without pausing	Evans Morris & Dunn Klein(1987)

Form 3.17: Normal EDS Development: Self-Feeding

Weeks of age	Skill
8–12 weeks	Makes small movements towards objects
12 weeks	Holds rattle placed in hand
16 weeks	Brings hands together in play
20 weeks	Approach movements begin. Mouths everything
24–28 weeks	Grasps. Will close palm around food and take to face. Bangs spoon. Shoulder control improving which helps in bringing spoon to mouth

Months of age	Skill
7–8 months	Holds bottle without help. Reaches towards dish. Picks up bits of food with thumb and first finger and takes to mouth
9–12 months	Offers but cannot release. Self-feeds defined lumps using thumb and forefinger. Drinks from cup held for him/her. Holds spoon but poor control
15 months	Finger-feeds well. Holds spoon with pronated grasp. Filling of spoon is poor. Spoon often overturns before reaching mouth
18 months	Fills spoon. Turns spoon in mouth, frequently spilling. Lifts cup to mouth bilaterally. May tip cup too much causing spilling. Beginning to release cup
24 months	Releases cup without spilling. Can hold small cup in one hand. Independent with spoon – moderate spillage. Spoon in mouth without turning
36 months	Little assistance needed. Beginning to use adult (supinated) grasp on utensils. Pours from jug. Uses fork
36–48 months	Spreads butter with knife
48–60 months	Cuts with knife

Based on Gessell (1940)

Form 3.18: Normal EDS Development Examples

Textures	0–6 months:	Liquids – breast/formula
	4–6 months:	Purées – bland, smooth, gluten-free (till 6 months) Winstock (1994) states 3–4 months
	8–12 months:	Mash, finger foods
	12–15 months:	Finely chopped
	15–24 months:	Table food (Evans Morris & Dunn Klein, 1987)
Food preferences	Birth:	Preference for sweet tastes, ie breast milk
	3 months:	Preference for other tastes
	6 months:	Preference for other tastes based on exposure to that taste
	1 year:	Preference for texture based on exposure to that food. Likes to imitate adults
	18 months:	Relative neophobia. Likes to imitate other children
	4 years:	Food categorisation complete. Has learned what can and cannot be eaten (Winstock, 1994)
Utensils	0–3 months:	Nipple/teat
	3–6 months:	Exposure to spoon feeding
	4–6 months/	
	6–9 months:	Cups/beakers introduced
	9–12 months:	Towards more adult spoon – more rigid, flatter bowl
	12–18 months:	Two-handled beaker
	18–36 months:	Open cup
	24–30 months:	Fork
	36–48 months:	Knife to spread butter
	48–60 months:	Knife to cut (Winstock, 1994)

Page 1 of 2

Form 3.18: *continued*

Food play	3–6 months:	Exploration through mouthing
	6–9 months:	Playing with food. Enjoys feeling food. Enjoys babbling with a mouthful of food
	9–12 months:	Enjoys playing with food – prodding, spreading, squeezing etc
	12–18 months:	Pretend play. Feeds self, others, toys
	24–60 months:	Plays with tea set, pots and pans. Helping adults in preparation
		Enjoys more elaborate pretend play such as shopping, cooking
		Enjoys helping to mix and stir (Winstock, 1994)
Behaviour & communication	9–12 months:	Shakes head for 'no'
	From 2–3 years:	Food refusal and fussiness are quite common
		Initial reaction to new foods is spitting out
	At 24–36 months:	Uses speech to express likes and dislikes

Form 3.19: Overview of the Developing Feeder

This section provides a developmental overview of children's eating and drinking, focusing on the global development rather than being skill-specific, and showing how EDS skills development 'fits' with this. It serves to reminds us how EDS skills are dependent on, and run concurrently with the development of other skills.

Carer task: Read through the handout and identify which stage most reflects your child's development.

Stage	Developmental stage	Age
1	Reflexive feeder	0–3 months
2	Developing feeder	4–6 months
3	Stabilising feeder	7–9 months
4	Controlled feeder	10–12 months
5	Refining feeder	13–15 months
6	Skill separation feeder	16–18 months
7	Independent feeder	19–24 months
8	Fine-tuner feeder	25–34 months

Reflexive feeder

- Primitive reflexes predominate
- No control (eg liquid loss)
- Jaw, tongue and lips do not move independently
- Position of physiological flexion.

Developing feeder

- Starts moving away from reflexive feeding – overrides primitive reflexes
- Gaining more stability in trunk/control
- Strong patterns still evident (eg tongue protrudes)
- Evidenced by changes in consistencies and utensils (eg purées, spoons)
- Starting self-feeding behaviours (eg hand to bottle).

Page 1 of 2

Form 3.19: *continued*

Stabilising feeder

■ Development of stability generally facilitates development of oral motor functions contributing to control in feeding. Evidenced by, for example finger feeding, controlled bite, opening mouth wide in anticipation of bolus

■ Still reduced control evidenced by, for example liquid loss on cups

■ Much greater combination of movements

■ Self-feeding more mature, for example assisting with spoon feeding.

Controlled feeder

■ Generally see overall control in feeding process, including structures such as jaw and less liquid loss

■ Gag less sensitive

■ Greater ability to move away from base of support.

Refining feeder

■ Generally stable physically and oral motorically, which gives opportunity to refine oral motor skills including, for example straw drinking and using teeth to remove food from spoon

■ No primitive patterns such as munching.

Skill separation feeder

■ Facilitates complex and complete movements – disassociation, for example midline transfer

■ Diagonal jaw movements

■ Good lip closure

■ Self-feeding with immature grip.

Independent feeder

■ All functions in place to facilitate independent feeding

■ End functions appear, for example using teeth to clean lip

■ No liquid loss.

Fine-tuner feeder

■ Details/movement options such as using tongue to clean lips, gums, cheek pockets

■ Increasing sensory awareness of taste and texture.

Page 2 of 2

Form 3.20: Goal Setting

1 **Encourage autonomy**. Develop independence through self-feeding. Move gradually towards shared control and planning meals with your child. The use of choices is sometimes appropriate, sometimes not. Graduated physical guidance can be given where necessary.

2 **Start with behaviour first**. Successful management of behaviour problems needs to be achieved before you can target eating skills. What behaviours should you target first? For example, learning to sit at the table?

3 **Take small steps**. Goals should be achievable and individualised. For example, if your child will not even smell food (never mind taste it) start with smelling first. Success is important, so set goals appropriately. It means the difference between success and failure. Moving too quickly can cause setbacks. Understand that change can be slow.

4 **Establish success for the goal** then increase the level of difficulty as appropriate. Progress towards the next goal.

5 **Manipulate only one variable at a time**, such as taste or texture

6 **Target behaviours need to be measurable**. They also need to be clearly defined so you can judge progress and ensure success. Keep accurate data and implement with precision. For example, don't say 'He must eat the whole bowl', state 'He will swallow five spoons of ...'. Be specific.

7 **Determine a maximum time limit**. In this approach, the time is not of consequence except to determine a maximum time limit. Children can use knowledge of a time limit to their advantage by not complying with goals. We have often extended sessions to fifty minutes or into the next EDS session before the children will comply. This may sound unnecessary, but when the child understands that refusal behaviour is not successful, such behaviour will decrease rapidly. Typically, children

Form 3.20: *continued*

who refuse over a lengthy time span do so only once or twice. They come to realise that the expectations of them remain unchanged and will then start to work with the carer co-operatively. However, a word of warning: with children with medical issues and oral motor dysfunction, always look out for signs of tiring. Safety first.

8 **Goals should be relevant to the child's developmental level**. For example, if a child has the developmental level of two years, but is chronologically five years old, goals should reflect the developmental level. This relates to having appropriate expectations of your child.

9 **Goals should follow a pattern of development**. For example, offer a new food in small quantities, then increase the volume of that food, then offer the next new food in small quantities, then increase the volume and so on.

10 **Provide a distraction-free environment**, especially if the child has a sensory disorder. This is a general guideline, as distraction can work well with some children.

11 **Use calming techniques** prior to feeding or do not lead up to meals with high-arousal activities. Also be neutral within the session.

12 **Give the child time to respond/comply**. Do not pressurise the child to perform quickly.

13 **Provide easy first goals**. On the first day, introduce textures and tastes that are not too challenging relative to the child. Provide experience of success.

14 **Model eating and drinking** when conducting EDS activities with the child. Don't expect your child to do what you will not.

15 **No negotiation**. Do not negotiate with the child regarding goals.

Form 3.20: *continued*

16 **Reinforcement should be provided** and decided upon pre-activity. It should not be given unless the goal is achieved but the reinforcement should not be withheld as a punishment, for example 'You were a bad boy, we are not going outside to the swings'. Instead, the child should be informed of non-achievement in neutral tones: 'Josh, you didn't take two bites of the biscuit'. The child needs to understand reinforcement is contingent upon achieving goals.

17 **No questions**. Never ask a child to meet the goals, tell the child in a firm but gentle manner that he is to meet them. Asking questions opens the route for refusal.

18 Likewise, **don't plead** for co-operation.

19 **Do not be tempted to change the rules** when things are going well. If the child does what you ask, reinforce and finish the session. Don't ask for 'one more spoon …' etc. The child needs to know you will not change the rules and are trustworthy.

20 **Be neutral** – your emotions should not be obvious in your face, voice or language.

21 **Restate goals as necessary** without doing so too frequently.

22 **Keep your focus**.

Page 3 of 3

Form 3.21: Carer Aims Sheet

Name of child _____   Date _____

Outline goals you have for you and your child for the Fun with Food programme:

1 _____
_____

2 _____
_____

3 _____
_____

4 _____
_____

5 _____
_____

Any other comments:

_____
_____
_____
_____
_____
_____
_____
_____
_____

Form 3.22: Staff Aims Sheet

Name of child _____   Date _____

Clinical staff _____

1 _____
_____

2 _____
_____

3 _____
_____

4 _____
_____

5 _____
_____

6 _____
_____

Identify priority goal

_____
_____
_____
_____
_____
_____
_____
_____

Form 3.23: Food for Thought Feedback Form

Please fill in the feedback form so we can adapt and improve the course in future. Your input and advice is much appreciated in making the programme better for carers, staff and children. Thank you for helping.

Please rate on a 1–5 scale where 1 = very poor, 2 = poor, 3 = okay/average,

4 = good, 5 = excellent

Activity	Rating	Comments
Interaction		
Nutrition		
Goal setting		
Feeding development		
Experiential eating		
Mealtime structure		
Most difficult thing		
Food memories		
Worst-case scenario		
Expectations		
Behaviour		
Therapy tips		

Other comments:

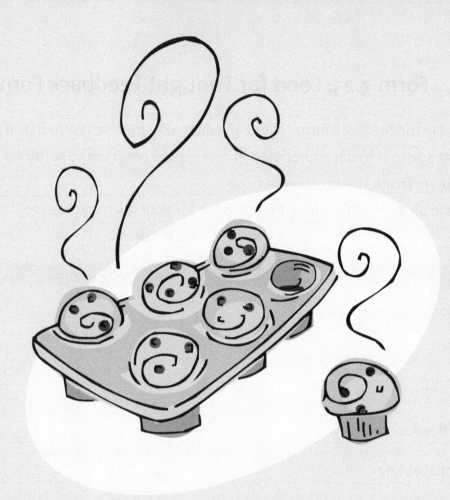

Chapter 4

STAGE 3

Fun before Food:
The pre-feeding programme

The Fun before Food element of the programme is the precursor to the Eating & Drinking & Swallowing section. Its overall aim is to prepare the child in particular, but also the carer, for actual EDS skills development. As noted in the introduction, it aspires to provide the foundation skills for oral feeding, develop readiness for oral feeding, and facilitate the development of a positive attitude to EDS.

This section contains session hints and activity suggestions for each element of the Fun before Food programme, that is:

- Growing Big & Strong
- Normalisation
- Food Play
- Oral Motor Skills
- Sensory Groups.

How long should Fun before Food run?

Children require time to carry over new skills learned and it is best to run this pre-feeding programme prior to (about two weeks before) the actual EDS element. The number of days this programme runs depends on the needs of the children and available resources, but 3–5 days should be the standard. Alternatively, it can be run on a weekly basis for one day a week.

ELEMENTS OF THE PROGRAMME

Staff guidelines

The handout Form 4.1 (see end of chapter), along with information sheets for each activity, is given to staff members involved in service provision in order to provide them with an overall view of the programme and their responsibilities within it.

Case notes

Case notes (Form 4.2) are, of course, useful for monitoring progress. In this programme they are doubly useful, given the number of different activities and activity leaders, and the intensity of the programme. A simple case note form can help activity leaders easily comply with record-keeping goals. There should be an identified location point both for masters (blanks) of the form and for completed copies, which can then be filed for the perusal of all involved.

The form allows for the following pieces of self-explanatory information to be recorded: child's name, session title (eg Normalisation), date, day number within the Fun before Food programme. Also included are:

- *Session goal*
  The goal tends to be broadly the same for each child within the group based on the activities designed for these sessions. However, depending on the developmental level of the child and the severity of the food aversion, more specific goals can often be set. For example, the activities for the first Normalisation session include exploring the sight and smell of different foods and symbolic play. However, it might be unrealistic to set these types of goal for a very aversive child, or a child who is still predominantly demonstrating exploratory rather than symbolic play, and so the goals can be adapted.

- *Outcome*
  The response of the child to each aspect of the activity is recorded with regard to how they approach and adapt to the activity, for what duration, what language/communication they engage in, and their general behaviour.

- *Action/Plan*
  This describes the action for the next session. However, within that it might include general recommendations regarding the next stage of the child's progress within a particular activity and, where appropriate, incorporate it into the next session. For example, an aversive child who only tolerates watching a carer take food out of a bag on the first day may allow the food to come a little closer or even be touched by it while it is still in its wrapper, the next time.

Eating & Drinking & Swallowing books

The EDS book sessions can be led by therapy assistants. Activity leaders should liaise with the staff member charged with running this session to ensure communication of homework goals. Homework activities develop or reinforce skills learned on the day and aim to encourage stabilisation or progression of that skill. Homework is directly related to the activities carried out on the day and typically involves an extension of that activity. The activities should reference the child's:

- developmental level
- level of aversion
- response to each individual activity within the session
- tolerance of activities in the activity/programme.

Each child is given an A5 scrapbook into which pictures, stickers and drawings can be added during this session. The scrapbook is called 'My Eating and Drinking and Swallowing Book'. Each activity conducted that day should have a separate page with the title of the activity on the top such as 'Food Play'. Suggested sentences to facilitate recall of the activity include: 'What I did today' and 'What I learned today'.

Useful materials for this activity include:

- Pictures
- Photographs (Polaroid or digital photographs taken during the day are useful for this activity)
- Stickers
- Symbols printed off a computer, for example from Boardmaker
- Catalogue picture cut-outs.

Each activity leader should ensure that they include homework materials in planning their sessions. A sample homework page might contain items such as those listed in Table 19.

As with all other activities, a handout (in this case Form 4.3) is given to carers prior to the first homework session, to explain the function and structure of the session.

Growing Big & Strong
Ger McGuirk

Inadequate nutrition has been recognised as a complication of both some types of disability (eg cerebral palsy) and EDS aversion. Luiselli (1989) states that the primary outcome of EDS aversion (whether selective or total) is chronic malnutrition and it is recognised that significant developmental progress can accompany improvements in nutritional status. The nutritional intake of children involved in the programme can be directly affected by a number of factors, including new foods, new textures, food temperature, food colour, eating away from home (eg school), the use of certain/different plates or cutlery, and the position of food on the plate. Sometimes these difficulties can come about as a result of the child's condition, for example Autistic

Spectrum Disorder can include a desire for order, increased oral sensory sensitivity, and a preference for familiar objects. Change imposed can often lead to confusion.

To encourage changes in eating habits, Fun with Food introduces healthy eating in a fun way where children (and carers) can learn about food and nutrition through play. Healthy eating can be discussed in a fun and non-threatening environment using toys (eg dolls) as the main characters, around which stories and activities are based. The aims of this element of the programme are to:

- Improve nutritional intake
- Heighten awareness of food and its nutritional content
- Broaden the range of food intake
- Introduce nutrient-dense food
- Prepare for the EDS element of the course.

Growing Big & Strong sessions are typically led by a dietitian, and are run each day of the Fun before Food programme, focusing on one to two food groups per day. (Some of these ideas are derived from the 'Teddy's Fun Food Pack' created by Epping Forest NHS.) These food groups are identified below and the handout Form 4.4 is given to parents with this information contained in it.

Big & strong foods: Foods that contain protein for growth and repair, such as meat, fish, eggs, beans, peas, lentils.
Teeth & bone foods: Foods that provide calcium for healthy bones and teeth, for example milk, cheese, yoghurt.

Table 19: Sample homework page

Session Title: Growing Big & Strong　　　　Date: _____

Today			
I	*(insert picture)*	**touched**	*(insert picture)*
Teddy	*(insert picture)*	**ate**	*(insert picture)*
Dolly	*(insert picture)*	**ate**	*(insert picture)*
Teddy	*(insert picture)*	**drank**	*(insert picture)*

Energy foods: Foods that give you energy, for example bread, potatoes, rice, breakfast cereals, pasta.

Helping-hand foods: Foods that contain vitamins, which are necessary for health. All fruits and vegetables (fresh, dried, tinned, frozen), fruit juice and vegetable juice.

Session hints

- The clinician should have a set of toys (teddies, dolls, miniature people, toy animals etc), but also encourage the child to bring his favourite toy to sessions, as this facilitates individualisation of information and goals, and encourages participation.
- Each of the four food groups is presented in separate containers, such as plastic storage boxes or wicker baskets. Real foods are utilised. Incorporate as many food varieties as possible. Make it look colourful and interesting. This encourages discussion among the carers and children. Ideas can be shared while the children play with the foods and become familiar with them.
- While foods can be offered to the carers and children, no pressure should be placed on children to eat at this stage of the programme. Carers, however, can model enjoyment of the smells and tastes of foods being discussed.
- Encourage the carer to use the Eating & Drinking & Swallowing book daily to record details of each session, and for homework purposes.

Activity suggestions

Activity 1: Big & strong foods
- Display slices of cooked ham, tins of sardines, tuna, salmon, cartons of eggs, tins of beans, peas and packets of lentils.
- Explain that these types of foods should be eaten each day as they are necessary for growth and repair. Show the child how these foods help him to grow big and strong by using the toys (eg when the doll hurts and cuts her leg, she needs to eat her meat and fish to make her better).
- Ask the child to suggest other big & strong foods.
- Facilitate a discussion on where we can buy big & strong foods ranging from uncooked varieties (supermarkets, butchers) to Fast Food outlets. What does the child prefer?
- Ask the child to suggest how they would use these foods in daily meal planning.
- Plan a main meal including foods on display.
- Cut out photographs of fish, chickens and eggs from magazines and paste into the Eating & Drinking & Swallowing book.

Activity 2: Teeth & bone foods

■ Use a container to display foods. Include cartons of milk, a variety of yoghurts (both smooth and fruit varieties), and a selection of cheeses. For the session to look more interesting include portions of cheeses cut into bite-size pieces (this may even encourage taste) and display the cheeses on colourful plates.

■ Use a display skeleton to initiate discussion on our bones. How many bones have humans? How many bones in our hands? Feet? Find the biggest bone. Find the longest one. What happens when bones break? Why are they important to us? What favourite activities can we do with our bones (eg run very fast, operate a see-saw, draw pictures)? What helps our bones grow from baby ones to tall adult ones?

■ Use pictures of different sets of teeth – preferably healthy and unhealthy representation. Include pictures of jaws with missing teeth. Use these to facilitate a discussion of teeth. Why are teeth useful? What do we do with them? What happens if we don't have them? How many teeth have each of the group (including the adults)?

■ Nutritional information can also be given, for example a glass of milk contains approx 220mg calcium, sufficient to meet one-third the needs of adults and children, and a cheese sandwich (45g) makes a substantial contribution to both adults' and children's daily needs of calcium and vitamins (McCance & Widdowson, 2002).

Activity 3: Energy foods

■ Display as many breads as possible in a basket along with pasta, rice and mini packets of breakfast cereals. Choose brown and white bread also pitta bread, fruit scones, brown scones.

■ Pasta in all shapes and colours attracts attention, so display in small bowls so that the children can run their fingers through them. All varieties of rice can also be displayed in small bowls.

■ Purchase and bake different breads with the child.

■ Display big and small and different kinds of potatoes.

Activity 4: Helping-hand foods

■ Display as many fruits and vegetables as possible. Choose exotic fruits like pineapple, mango, kiwi, passion fruit and so on. Fruit and vegetables should be fresh and crispy. Have some fruits cut up and displayed on small plates. Use tinned as well as fresh varieties.

■ Select a variety of fruits and vegetables and a big world map and facilitate a brainstorming activity on the country of origin of each piece of fruit and vegetable. Retain labels on purchased fruit and vegetables for this activity.

■ Make smoothies (and suggest the use of fruit and yoghurt in a smoothie drink).

- Get the child to assist in making a homemade soup by helping to cut up foods if appropriate (and under carer guidance), or place pre-cut up foods into soup dishes/pots.
- Draw pictures of vegetables and fruits (eg carrots and tomatoes). What colour should they be?
- Facilitate a discussion on why humans need energy and where we get it from. Present a range of normal activities, such as from sleeping to racing, and get the child to use a rating scale for the energy required to carry out each activity. Use visual representations, for example from a tiny pebble-sized bit of energy to mountainfuls of energy.
- Get the child to draw favourite fruits and vegetables.

Additional Growing Big & Strong suggestions incorporating the four food groups

- Stories centred around the 'dolly's/teddy's day' (from breakfast to supper) can be told using a cardboard poster or flip-chart paper. Boardmaker symbols can be used to create charts with options and choices such as breakfast foods. Alternatively, cut out labels or use real packs. Stimulate discussion by asking, for example:
  – What does dolly/teddy have for breakfast?
  – What do you have?
  – Is dolly/teddy sitting with her family at the table? etc.
  Continue with the story to include both lunch and supper.
- Involving the child in a pretend picnic is an easy way to incorporate the four food groups. For example:
  – Ask the child to make a sandwich using food from the baskets.
  – What yoghurt will we bring? Which basket was it in?
  – Would dolly/teddy like a piece of fruit?
  – What would dolly/teddy have to drink?
- Posters can be made by the children and coloured in.
- Cut-out pictures of foods and empty food boxes can be used in playing shop. Use baskets and pretend money/checkouts and so on.
- Make food out of play dough.
- A 'What I ate diary' can be made or the EDS homework books used. Ask the child what he ate for breakfast (older children could keep a diary), and encourage use of pictures or colouring. Underline the different food groups in different colours for emphasis, encouraging the children to identify, for example, 'Which food is an energy food?'

Normalisation

Damhnait Ní Mhurchú

Normalisation refers to activities to do with food that don't actually involve eating and drinking. The interpretation of normalisation adopted for the purposes of the Fun before Food programme covers involvement in play around the rituals of eating and drinking, including an extension of food play and exposure to the broader context of habits and tasks relating to food, drink and mealtimes in general. The approach adopted to introduce Normalisation follows a developmental framework, and predominantly incorporates play in pursuit of activities.

When dealing with children who have difficulty with, or have aversion to, EDS it is easy to exclude them from the rituals and behaviours around eating because they may not be involved in the actual activity itself. Recognition of this exclusion through actively engaging children in these activities in a treatment programme is twofold. First, it is another stage in building their child's confidence in approaching food without the threat of having to eat it, and second, it is also an opportunity for these children to experience and participate in activities from which they are otherwise potentially excluded.

Mealtimes and food preparation are all learning opportunities as well as frequently being family time. Copeland and Kimmel (1989) discuss how dinnertime provides an opportunity for the whole family to reinforce skills in the areas of social, language and motor skills. Mealtimes are times when children interact with the rest of the family, learn about food, learn from helping to prepare food and cleaning up and generally experience structures and predictable routines (Klein & Delaney, 1994).

Apart from the immediate consequences to the food-aversive child of exclusion from normalisation activities, there is also a ripple effect, which can extend from immediate carers, to siblings, across extended family and even the community, caused by the child's difficulty in participating in a wide range of routine and celebratory events that involve food. We know that the purpose of eating and drinking is not mere survival but has socio-cultural significance. Routines such as mealtimes, either everyday or special events, allow for group cohesion (Case-Smith, 2001). Such normal activities as food shopping, going to coffee shops or restaurants or attending birthday parties are not within the usual scope of experience of the child with EDS aversion.

The inclusion of normalisation in the Fun before Food programme begins to address this imbalance of experience on the part of the child and recognises the non-nutritional effects of an aversive feeding difficulty from the perspective of the whole family.

The research is plentiful in detailing the developmental acquisition of eating and drinking skills; however, Copeland and Kimmel (1989) refer to the pattern of eating *behaviours* of typically developing children, and it is important to consider what is appropriate at a particular developmental stage regarding the *preparation* and *anticipation* of eating and drinking activities. McInnes and Treffney (1982) describe the hierarchy of development of skills around mealtime preparation of initially pouring liquid from a jug into a cup or bowl, setting the table, clearing the table and building up to the most complex skill of washing up.

Once the developmental level of the child has been established, activities can be introduced through play as children learn to integrate sensory, motor, cognitive, perceptual and social skills, and learn about their world through play (Doyle Morrison & Metzger, 2001). Play also offers us the 'cultural contexts' to organise behaviours for particular reasons (Vandenberg & Kielhofner, 1982). These are cornerstones in the Fun with Food approach.

A recurring theme in the research, though, is the importance of the role of context, and this too is important in the practical application of the Fun with Food approach. The focus in Normalisation is not just on the child, but also recognising the importance of carers, siblings, the extended family and the child's environment. Consequently, any activities adopted in this area need to be meaningful, practical and cognizant of the everyday reality of the child's life. Setting the table is meaningful only for the child and his family who eat at a table.

The specific aims of the Normalisation sessions are to:

■ Provide experience of food in a non-threatening environment
■ Provide the child and their carer(s) with experience of food and food-related activities other than eating
■ Extend the child's knowledge and experience of food.

Session hints

■ Seat each child at tables around the treatment room and provide them with materials
■ Seat children near or apart from the others depending on their developmental level
■ Do not force a child to engage in any activity that they are defensive about.

Activity suggestions

Activity 1: Feely bag
A feely bag activity to explore food with the senses of touch and smell in particular. Suggested foods include:

- Taste/Smell:
  - Sour: concentrated lemon juice
  - Spicy: tomato paste/ketchup
  - Sweet: a sip drink, jelly tots
  - Bland: plain biscuits, fromage frais
  - Fishy: Worcestershire sauce
- Textures:
  - Hard: biscuit
  - Soft: marshmallow
  - Smooth: apple
  - Sticky: dates
  - Greasy: puffed crisps
  - Wet: yoghurt
  - Furry: peach
  - Textured: rice, hundreds-and-thousands.

Many foods will address a number of different areas (eg a plain biscuit will be both bland and hard, a peach will be sweet smelling and tasting, but furry to touch).

The idea here is for initial food exposure and exploration. Offer children the opportunity to look at, feel, smell and, if the child initiates it, taste different foods. Presenting the foods in a feely bag is not only a fun way of finding out about them, but also means that if the child feels particularly threatened by this exposure to food, the bag offers some security by being a barrier they can elect to overcome. Encourage children to look at and explore the feely bag both verbally and through modelling.

Activity 2: Pretend tea party
A pretend teddy and dolly tea party using toys but with access to real food.

This will offer the child the opportunity to experience food without the threat of having to eat it, and also give them the experience of playing out the rituals of mealtime through pretend play as a 'prelude to reality'. For the child for whom it is developmentally appropriate to engage in symbolic play, model feeding dolly and teddy while labelling and expanding on the activity. Vocabulary should be food-centred, focusing on textures, smells etc.

Activity 3: Go to the shop

A visit to a local supermarket to purchase food with a view to cooking and preparing it later. Extra time should be built into the timetable for such an external activity. An outing to a supermarket is a very normal, typical activity for the majority of children, but perhaps not for the child with aversion. The visit itself also exposes the child to food and drink outside of the context of actually having to eat it.

Choose a supermarket a short distance from where treatment is taking place. Provide some money to the carer and child team for purchases, but do not limit the value of purchases. Advise carers to purchase food items that could be prepared or 'cooked' in the clinic the next day with relative ease, such as prepared puddings.

Activity 4: Let's cook!

This is the preparation and cooking of food purchased the previous day in the supermarket. This activity exposes the child to food, physically touching food, and food preparation, in a non-threatening way. It also increases control over the food in question as the child prepares the food himself or is an active participant in the process. Initially, the child and the carer should prepare for 'cooking' by setting the table and fetching necessary utensils and crockery. Most families choose packet dessert mixes that only need to be whisked with milk, and take turns in ripping the packets open, spilling out the contents into a bowl and stirring. The activity can be expanded on for those who are developmentally ready by decorating newly prepared desserts with jellies, hundreds-and-thousands, chocolate buttons and so on. This allows for a smooth transition from Normalisations to Food Play sessions when timetabled after one another.

As suggested above, it is inappropriate to set teddy's food party activities for a child who is still predominantly at an exploratory play level, or play restaurant games with a child with very limited language skills. Equally, it is unrealistic to expect a child who is only beginning to tolerate the presence and smell of food to actively decorate cakes. It is important, when setting up homework activities for the individual child, to set them up within a graded hierarchical system allowing for increasing complexity of activity and increasing hands-on involvement by the child himself. It is also important to attempt to cover a range of Normalisation activities that reflect the different aspects of this area, and the approach taken. Consequently, homework activities, while structured within a developmental framework and tailored to the individual needs of the child, should be introduced through play *and* normal everyday activities, and be socio-culturally appropriate.

Additional suggestions for homework activities which can be built into the daily routine are listed in Table 20.

Some of the activities mentioned are adapted and expanded on from Klein and Delaney (1994). Carers can be given Form 4.6 to help with carrying out homework. The handout explaining rationale and structure of this session (Form 4.5) is given to carers at the start of the first session.

Table 20: Normalisation homework activities

Activity	Homework suggestions
Cooking	There are a lot of ready-prepared items in supermarkets which make cooking easy for the child, including bread and buns, prepared desserts, dips and sauces etc
Sensory immersion	Each day choose between two and four different foods to explore by vision, touch and smell Contrast and compare
Equipment	Select equipment associated with food such as appliances, crockery, utensils, shops, rooms etc Compare and contrast uses and colours
Play	Tea parties (with and without food) Playing restaurant Playing shop Pretend meals at home
Experience of mealtime rituals	Food preparation Table setting/preparation of required utensils Clearing away Washing up Putting away/emptying out dishwasher
Exposure to/ participation in everyday activities	Going to supermarket/different food shops Helping with shopping lists Going out to coffee shops/restaurants Organising/attending parties etc.

Food Play

Trish Morrison

The reason for the food play activity is to desensitise children to, and provide fun experience with, different textured foods in a non-threatening and supportive environment. The aims therefore include the following:

■ To desensitise the child to food smells and textures
■ To help prepare the child for eating
■ To assist in developing a positive attitude to food.

By the age of two months an infant is already gathering sensory information and integrating it, establishing the foundation for future learning. The tactile sense is the primary source of information and learning, where touch generally feels pleasant on the skin and in and around the mouth, and eating provides positive feedback (Stock Kranowitz, 1998).

Increasing numbers of children are surviving prematurity and other neonatal complications, and they can present with long histories of invasive oral procedures, one of which is tube feeding. Consequently, they may miss out on critical periods of oral exploration and weaning, which can result in hypersensitivity and limited or no positive food experiences. A child with tactile dysfunction may:

■ Avoid touching certain textures or surfaces
■ Avoid messy play
■ Be a picky eater
■ Avoid particular food textures (Stock Kranowitz, 1998).

Food play must always be conducted within a supportive, relaxed environment, and the clinician must remember to:

> dance on the edge of tolerance or the treatment will not be effective in making a change. *(Wolf & Glass, 1992)*

Guidelines for food play activities include:

■ Food play should be goal-directed, appropriate to the child's level of food play, non-directive and fun, supervised by an adult, and designed to encourage but not force the child to explore and, where possible, taste food.

- Food textures chosen for use during food play should be appropriate to the child's oral motor skills if it is possible that the food will be tasted.
- Food should be tasted from the knuckles first as these cannot go so far into the child's mouth, hence there is less risk of gagging.
- Allow mess; indeed, a certain amount of mess should be encouraged and is the hallmark of a successful session.
- Ensure the child is comfortable with all levels of food play prior to focusing on eating.

As for all activities, carers attend with the child and participate actively. Carers should be provided with a copy of the Food Play handout (Form 4.9), which can be found at the end of this chapter.

In Fun before Food a developmental approach to the levels of food play is used. While each child is approached as an individual, these stages help to inform where to begin therapy and what to try next. The child progresses through the broad categories listed in Table 21.

Table 21: Categories of food play progression

Stage	Explanation
Pretend food play	Seen as a foundation upon which more advanced skills develop, that is, dry and finally wet food play
Dry food play	Divided into stages representing developmental progress. A child progresses from coarse to increasingly fine dry textures
Wet food play	Divided into stages representing developmental progress. The development relates to the type of tactile feedback the child gets from the food. Generally it is our experience that a child progresses through the following stages in wet food play: Wet firm consistencies Wet tacky consistencies Wet semi-solid consistencies Wet liquid consistencies Wet mixed textures.

Session hints

1 Set up a separate play area for each family with materials for the activity in a central location. This enables each child to work on a food play activity suitable to their individual needs.

2 Sessions should have a predictable beginning (putting on aprons and gathering materials) and end (clearing the table and washing hands).

3 The goals and rationale within food play should be written specifically for each child. These should, as with all therapy goals, be specific and attainable; however, the general goals and rationale remain unchanged regardless of the level of food play focused on.

4 Experience tells us that children who are comfortable with all levels of food play prior to commencing the EDS element of the programme make the transition to oral eating more easily. It is worth investing considerable time and effort in this area from the outset.

5 The pretend food play level is usually completed relatively easily, within the first session, with longer periods of time being needed for dry and wet food play.

6 Many of the activities suggested in the pretend food play section can be adapted to become dry and wet food play games by substituting real foods of the appropriate textures.

7 Many children find it difficult to progress from dry to wet food play; this transition can be facilitated with a little ingenuity, for example:
   (a) Create a barrier between the child's hand and the wet food, for example by manipulating ketchup and mayonnaise to make pink when both foods are held within a zip-lock bag.
   (b) Allow the child to use surgical gloves initially for food painting, gradually reducing the barrier by cutting some of the fingers from the gloves or only covering one finger with a finger toothbrush (Stock Kranowitz, 1998).

8 Any of the activities can be adapted to a level of exploratory play with utensils (spoons/cups) or hands according to learning level.

9 While the overall aim is to move through each of the three major food textures, individual aims for each child need to be pitched according to their tolerance and success within each session in addition to their level of learning. For example, work through levels of coarseness of dried foods over Fun before Food programme days for the less tolerant child.

Activity suggestions

Activity suggestions are listed in Table 22.

Table 22: Food play activities

Activity	Aim	Equipment	Play suggestions
Exposure to dry food	Exposure to dry food materials through games/activities working down through levels of coarseness	Dried butter-beans, dried chickpeas, hard sweets, lentils and medium-coarseness maize Toy cars, trucks	Driving toy cars/trucks through various dried foods of different coarseness Running hands through trays of dried food Scooping beans, lentils, etc from one tray to another Sticking lentils, maize, etc to card to make a 'picture'
Exposure to wet food materials	Exposure to wet food materials through games/activities working down through levels of tackiness to thinner consistencies	Jelly (made up from packet), treacle, chocolate spread, yoghurt Plastic animals	Cutting out jelly shapes, scooping jelly in and out of containers Finger painting with treacle, chocolate spread, etc on card Plastic animals playing in 'swamp' created from above material
Exposure to mixed wet and dry food materials	Exposure to mixed wet and dry food materials through games/activities working down through the levels of coarseness and consistency	Treacle, chocolate spread, yoghurt and sweets, hundreds-and-thousands, cooked cold spaghetti and biscuits Paper plates Plastic animals	Create a face on a paper plate with the different materials such as yoghurt for skin, spaghetti for hair, sweets for features etc Develop the 'swamp' theme with plastic animals/dinosaurs moving from sandy (maize) areas to sticky areas (chocolate spread/treacle) etc 'Build' houses, etc by sticking together biscuits as bricks using the wet textures

continued

Table 22: *continued*

Activity	Aim	Equipment	Play suggestions
Pretend food play	To touch items such as cutlery and cooking utensils To engage in short periods of pretend play (specify a time) To be comfortable with pretend food play, food utensils and packaging prior to engaging with food directly	Pretend toys and foods Bowls Picnic baskets, empty food containers Toy fruit or vegetable tins, chocolate money scented gel pens, card for price tags scented gel pens Feely bag, kitchen utensils	*Pretend tea parties for dolls, teddies, and carers:* Make pretend sandwiches, pour out crisps, sweets, etc into bowls *Pretend teddy bears' picnic:* Pack a picnic, use real picnic baskets and empty food containers *Pretend shop:* Set up different sections of a supermarket using fruit or vegetable tins, bakery, etc. Then play shop and include chocolate or rice paper money or scented gel pens to make price tags and other signs *Restaurant:* Talk about a menu, prepare the room, set the tables and pretend to prepare the food, using real utensils, then pretend to cook and serve it. You could use scented gel pens to prepare the menu. *Feely bag:* Blindfold the children if they are happy with this, dip a hand into a container and select a kitchen utensil, examine it and guess what it is

continued →

Table 22: *continued*

Activity	Aim	Equipment	Play suggestions
Dry food play	To touch and play with food for brief periods; the timescale will be established for each child individually by the clinician. This goal may need to be subdivided allowing for increasing time periods. The activities enable the child and carer to become comfortable exploring foods using a variety of senses, touch, smell and possibly taste. Within dry food play the child is exposed to different textured dry foods progressing from coarse foods, eg cereals or porridge, to increasingly fine foods, such as polenta and flour	Different textured dry foods progressing from coarse foods, eg cereals or porridge, to increasingly fine foods such as polenta and flour Barrel Trays Glue	*Jewellery and accessory making* with dry foods of an appropriate texture: eg bracelets, necklaces, bandanas or belts. Use ring-shaped dry foods such as savoury snacks, sweets and cereals, as well as pasta and popcorn *Food fights*: Engage in flinging dry foods around – this could resemble a snow ball or pillow fight! Use rice, pasta, dried beans, lentils and, if you are very brave, flour. Obviously, ensure that no one gets hurt or injured! *Lucky dips*: Hide novelty items in a barrel containing dried foods of an appropriate texture *Art & crafts*: Use trays to help contain the foods. Apply glue to a page then blow hundreds-and-thousands around the page to make a pattern. Use other dried foods of an appropriate texture, eg if working on fine dry foods include herbs, spices and flours *Food pictures*: Use pasta, popcorn, cereal, pieces of crumbled biscuits, flours, herbs and spices to make food collages, apply glue to the page and then add the food *Food walk*: Put out dried foods on a tray then 'take your finger for a walk'. Play follow-the-leader with the clinician

continued ➜

Table 22: *continued*

Activity	Aim	Equipment	Play suggestions
Dry food play *continued*		Different textured dry foods progressing from coarse foods, eg cereals or porridge, to increasingly fine foods such as polenta and flour	*Cookery:* These activities overlap with Normalisation activities. Make recipes that require the use of dried foods, eg crunching the biscuits for a cheesecake base, taking out handfuls of cereals to make buns. *Imaginative play:* Make characters walk through, dive into, jump, run, swim or roll in a tray of dried food. This could take the format of a 'Simon Says' game
Wet food play	To touch and play with food of the target texture for a brief period. The activities enable the child and carer to become comfortable exploring wet food using a variety of senses such as touch, smell and possibly taste	Plastic animals, model people, toy cars, trucks	*Building:* Model villages or farm using a cereal mixed with water for muddy fields, or soil in a pretend garden, jelly set in moulds for the buildings, lollipops for signposts, strips of liquorice or cooked pasta to mark the roads, rivers of cream or coloured water. Move animals or model people around the village or farm, across rivers etc. *Dirt tracks:* Build a dirt track with jelly for hills, cereal mixed with water for mud, rivers of custard or yoghurt, swamps of rice pudding etc. Drive vehicles through the course, beginning with large vehicles, progressing to small ones as the child is ready to have more contact with the different food textures
		Make-up brushes chocolate or strawberry sauce	*Make-up/face painting:* Apply make-up to dolls or willing carers of the children! Use different brushes as applicators. Invent strawberry or chocolate sauce lipstick, or eye shadows

continued →

Table 22: *continued*

Activity	Aim	Equipment	Play suggestions
Wet food play *continued*	To touch and play with food of the target texture for a brief period. The activities enable the child and carer to become comfortable exploring wet food using a variety of senses such as touch, smell and possibly taste		*Cookery:* This is an area where food play overlaps with Normalisation activities, the difference being that within food play the recipe chosen should reflect the level of wet food play being targeted. Examples are given below
		Different coloured food sauces	*Food painting:* Finger painting with food, eg sauces. Include mixing foods to make new colours, eg ketchup and mayonnaise to make pink!
		Brushes	*Splatter painting:* Apply the food to a brush and then splatter on a page
		Food colouring, cornflour	*Cornflour painting:* Mix the cornflour with water to a creamy consistency; add food colouring or essences as desired. Place each colour in a shallow dish and paint, including finger painting
		Fruit and vegetables	*Fruit and vegetable prints:* Cut a fruit or vegetable in half and sculpt out a shape, dip the shape in food or paint and print on paper.

Within wet food play, work through the categories of food outlined in Table 23. The clinician may need to begin with bland foods if the child has difficulty tolerating food smells.

For the final session carers are responsible for planning a food play session appropriate to their child's needs.

Food Play Chart (Form 4.8)

Use Form 4.8 to chart and monitor the child's progress through Food Play sessions. For directions for use, see the sample Food Play Chart (Form 4.7) at the end of the chapter.

- Record the child's name and the date of the sessions in the spaces provided
- Note the type of food used
- Record the level of food play on which the child is working using the key provided
- Describe the child's responses
- Note the next target level of food play in the action column.

Table 23: Wet food hierarchy

Consistency	Example	Suggested activity
Wet firm	Dough	Make pizza dough, bread or scones
Wet tacky	Cooked rice pasta	Make fruit crumble
Wet semi-solid	Set custard Greek yoghurt Jelly Mousse	Make Angel Delight, jelly or mousse
Liquids	Pouring custard Pouring cream Yoghurts	Make pancake batter or juices
Mixed textures	Minestrone soup Pasta and sauce Rice pudding Pizza with a topping	Make pizza toppings, krispie buns or fruit salad

Oral Motor Skills

Petro Van Deventer

> It is essential to provide a diversity of oral motor opportunities with various options for sensory input and motoric response because the motor requirements to accommodate different textures, sizes, shapes, temperatures and tastes drive oral motor development. *(Boshart, 1998)*

The main aim of this section of the Fun with Food approach centres around building the foundation for the development of more refined oral motor skills. In order to understand and perform a skill, the child needs to know how it works, and learn the underlying skills. This can be so daunting and demanding that the child may feel reluctant or even fearful to try it. By starting at a level where the child feels confident that he can achieve success, the clinician can help him begin the journey of building a positive attitude towards his oral area.

The starting point is to increase a child's oral facial awareness through improved knowledge of the different parts of the face and mouth, and their functions. If the child becomes more familiar with his mouth and how different sensations feel, the exploration of various textures, shapes and movements in the mouth become less threatening and more comfortable as he starts to make sense of what he experiences. The mouth is no longer just one big area where every sensation is blurred and almost painfully unfamiliar. Touch and movement become more refined and localised, and in the process more meaningful.

> Orally defensive children perceive the mouth as a whole – one continuous kinaesthetic area ... therefore sensation is muddled and differentiation is blocked. *(Marshalla, 2001)*

By using a very graded and gradual approach, the clinician can guide the child towards accepting touch on the face and inside the mouth.

Once this has been achieved the child is then encouraged to engage in oral imitation tasks to introduce and familiarise themselves with the different movements of each oral structure. Oral motor tools can be used to facilitate and refine skills, and to encourage oral exploration in a non-threatening environment. As activities are devised to meet the sensory needs of clients, children feel more in control and are therefore more willing to engage in activities to achieve the ultimate goal of developing the strength, mobility and co-ordination of movement required for effective eating and drinking. The handout on oral motor skills (Form 4.12) can be found at the end of the chapter.

Oral Motor Record Form (Form 4.10)

Each session has a general goal as stated in the session plans. Within each session the child is introduced to various tasks. When making observations of a child's performance, behaviour should be documented in terms of oral facial awareness, response to touch, ability to imitate and explore oral movements demonstrated, as well as ability to perform the oral motor tasks introduced. The initial oral motor goals for each child should be documented after the assessment of each child.

The session form (Form 4.10) should be completed as follows:

1 Document the general goal of the session
2 Specify individual goals for each child according to their abilities
3 Indicate whether the child reached his goals and, if not, document details regarding specific behaviour observed
4 State the plan/goal for the next session.

For an example of this see Table 24.

Session hints

1 It is important to:
   ■ Explain to the child what you are doing
   ■ Share information
   ■ Be specific and consistent
   ■ Use firm pressure
   ■ Work from the least to the most sensitive area
   ■ Use puppets and music.
2 On the face, go from the cheeks to the jaw to around and on the lips. Tools used can range from the gloved hand, soft puppet, wash cloth to vibrator.
3 Inside the mouth, go from the gums/teeth to inside the cheeks to the surface of tongue, tongue blade and lateral margins of the tongue, to the palate. Tools used can range from NUK®, toothette, toothbrush, clinician's finger and Infadent.

Table 24: Sample oral motor goals

Example	Goal status	Goal/Achievement
Example A	General goal:	Increased awareness of the face and mouth
	Specific goals for A:	Oral facial awareness: to be able to identify his lips
	Achieved goal:	Yes
	Next step:	Identify teeth
Example B	General goal:	Response to touch
	Specific goals for B:	Tolerate touch around the lips
	Achieved goal:	Yes
	Next step:	Tolerate touch on the lips
Example C	General goal	Imitation tasks
	Specific goals for C:	To round lips
	Achieved goal:	No. Very little movement
	Next step:	Repeat activity, provide tactile cue
Example D	General goal:	Oral motor tasks
	Specific goals for D:	Breathe on bubble caught on wand
	Achieved goal:	Yes
	Next step:	Blow bubble off the bubble wand
		(Bubble-blowing hierarchy: Rosenfeld-Johnson, 2001)

4 On oral exploration tasks:
   - Encourage exploration
   - Vary methods
   - Normalise tactile sensitivity
   - Explore together
   - Show/demonstrate ways
   - Talk about movement
   - Describe and label.

Tools used can range from horns/whistles, toothbrushes, tongue depressors, bite blocks, Chewy Tubes, NUK®, straws and tubing (see Tools & Resources sections).

Activity suggestions

These are listed in Tables 25 to 27.

Table 25: Oral motor activities 1

Activity 1: My face and mouth

Rationale

To gain confidence in the exploration of oral movements, children need to be aware of the different parts of their face and mouth, and the movements these structures are capable of.

Goal

Children will become more aware of the different parts of their face and explore different oral facial movements.

Preparation for the session

Draw, cut out and laminate different parts of a face, eg eyes, ears, nose, mouth, hair, eyebrows.
Draw a large oval shape on a blank piece of paper. This will serve as a face.
Take photographs of all the children attending the group (this can be done on Assessment Day).
Draw, cut out and laminate the different parts of the mouth. Include the following: lips, tongue, teeth, soft palate.
Cut out pictures of different facial expressions from magazines.

A. Building a face

Position the paper with the oval shape against a wall where it is visible to all the children. The clinician and the more able children can take turns to stick different facial features on the oval shape, one at a time.
After each part is named and positioned on the oval, carers assist their child in locating the particular feature on his own face. The use of a mirror will contribute to the success of the activity. Encourage the child to look at his own facial expressions in the mirror. The clinician requests children to look at pictures of different facial expressions and to copy them.

B. What do I look like?

Place the photographs taken before the session in a feely bag. Each child gets a turn to take a photograph from the bag and identify who is on the picture by either pointing to or stating the name of the specific child. The different features as well as the facial expression of each child are discussed, eg eye colour, wearing spectacles etc.

continued →

Table 25: *continued*

Activity 1: My face and mouth

C. What is inside my mouth?

Repeat the earlier parts of activity 1. This time use the laminated parts of the inside of the mouth. Encourage the child to point to, touch or move the different parts of their mouth as each oral structure is discussed. For example, when discussing:

■ The lips: encourage opening and closing of the mouth/blow a kiss etc.

■ The teeth: encourage counting of teeth, bite down or clatter teeth

■ The tongue: demonstrate different tongue movements and encourage copy of these (eg protrusion, elevation)

End the session by introducing the adventures of Mr Tongue or Mouth Madness (see Tools & Resources) mouth rhymes to practise different movements.

D. Homework

Summary of oral structures discussed during the session. Use Boardmaker symbols. As revision, carers help their child to paste pictures in homework books of all the different parts of the face and mouth the child saw, touched and moved today.

In the mirror, encourage the child to look at himself to touch and move different parts of the face and mouth.

Table 26: Oral motor activities 2

Activity 2: All the things I can do with my mouth

Rationale

Exploring the mouth and its movements in a pleasurable way is an unfamiliar experience for a child with aversive feeding behaviour. With the introduction of oral toys, this experience can be fun and interesting.

Goal

Children will engage in a variety of oral motor and oral imitation tasks within their sensory needs.

Preparation for the session

Collect items for blowing and oral exploration such as horns, whistles, ping-pong balls, feathers, cut-out fish/animal shapes from tissue paper, plastic insects etc.

Collect items for biting such as tubing, Chewy Tubes, straws, spatulas etc.

Collect items for licking and exploration such as spoons, stamps, envelope, spatulas etc.

Children sit in a circle with their carers and the clinician. Each child and their carer share a hand mirror.

A. My lips

In the first part of the activity, engage in oral imitation tasks to explore all the different movements of the lips, eg smiling, kissing, lip rounding (for blowing and sucking).

During the second part of the activity, oral tools are used to touch the lips and to practise blowing. Use items mentioned in the preparation section. Each child gets a box with tools for blowing and can choose which tool they want to use first. It is helpful to sit the child in front of a mirror so that the child can watch the movement of his lips. Carers give feedback to children and encourage experimentation with all toys for a short while.

If a child is not ready to cope with the handling/manipulation of oral tools, observing a carer or peers engaging in and enjoying oral motor activities can be beneficial.

continued ➔

Table 26: *continued*

Activity 2: All the things I can do with my mouth

B. My teeth

In the first part of the activity, children and carers engage in oral imitation tasks to become more aware of what they can do with their teeth, such as pretending to bite or chew. Children are shown that they can see their teeth when they smile and they can use their lips to hide their teeth.

Then children are encouraged to bite down and look at their teeth, while holding a smiling posture. A puppet is introduced to demonstrate biting and chewing on oral tools and imitation is encouraged. Children who are not ready to use oral tools themselves are prompted to let a puppet bite/chew on a tool of their choice. Use tools mentioned in the preparation section. During the next activity, children and their carers pretend to be puppies and engage in tugging games with straws.

Pretend to be cats and use straws for whiskers. Children have to bite down on straws to keep them in place. Use puppets to perform these tasks if children are not yet ready to engage in these games themselves.

C. My tongue

In the first part of this activity, children and their carers engage in oral imitation tasks to explore different movements of the tongue, including licking, elevation and lateralisation. They are encouraged to use their tongues to touch different places inside their mouths such as teeth, inside of the cheek, roof of the mouth etc.

Then children use different objects to explore with their tongue and to practise licking. Use items mentioned in the preparation section.

D. Homework

Summary of session. Use Boardmaker symbols: these are all the things I can do with my mouth. Choose appropriate items for each child according to the specific activities they participated in. Paste in their homework books. For example:

- I can bite and chew: (Chewy Tubes, tubing, ice-cream sticks, straw, toothbrush)
- I can lick: (my lips, my fingers, a spoon, a stamp, an ice-cream stick)
- With my lips I can: (blow, kiss, smile, suck)

Practise Mr Tongue adventures at home.

Table 27: Oral motor activities 3

Activity 3: Exercises just for me!

Rationale

Through the introduction of specific activities, the strength, mobility and co-ordination of movement in a child's oral structures can be improved. These skills take time to develop and require frequent repetition.

Goal

Children will engage in activities devised to meet their specific needs, to ultimately improve their foundation skills for feeding.

Preparation for the session

Use information obtained from the Assessment Day and clinical observation to devise a sensory oral motor programme specific to each child's needs.

Key-workers discuss and demonstrate individual sensory motor programmes to carers. Each child is presented with a goodie bag containing oral toys suitable to meet his individual needs as identified on the Assessment Day and through clinical observations made during the first two days of the Fun before Food programme. Guidelines given in this programme have to be followed regularly until the start of the EDS component of the programme.

Example A: Oral facial awareness

Photographs: collect photographs from magazines and use Polaroid or digital photographs of the children.

Mirror work: use a mirror to copy facial expressions. Encourage children to imitate tongue, lip and jaw movements.

Rhymes and song: focus on specific parts of the face and mouth in a song or use the face and mouth to act out rhymes.

Puppets: identify different parts of the face/mouth on a puppet. Encourage children to find the same facial features on their own faces.

Naming: name different parts of the face and mouth during daily routines.

Example B. Normalisation to touch

Use touch appropriate to the child's level of sensitivity, and work from the least to the most sensitive areas. The same sequence is followed every time, moving very slowly towards the ultimate goal of tolerance or even enjoyment of oral facial stimulation.

Tools that can be suggested for use on the face include the gloved hand, soft puppet, wash cloth, vibrator.

Tools that can be suggested for use inside the mouth include the gloved finger, toothbrush, NUK® brush, Infadent, toothette.

continued ➜

Table 27: *continued*

Activity 3: Exercises just for me!

Example C: Oral exploration

The child develops a variety of motor plans for different textures, shapes and sizes introduced by mouthing appropriate toys. For example, a child who has difficulty coping with lumpy foods may benefit from experiences with non-food items with characteristics similar to the food items avoided. Tools are explored and shared with the child before approaching their face. Discuss all the different features of each tool – texture, shape, colour etc. Add language to the experience by describing what the child is experiencing. Guide the child to explore oral toys in different ways. For example, if they only chew on a tool, perhaps they can slide their tongue over the surface etc.

Tools for exploration include horns, tubing, plastic foods, toothbrush, NUK® brush, straws etc.

Example D: Oral motor activities

Tools are introduced to target specific skills. These exercises have to be repeated over a period of time to develop strength and co-ordination of movements. For example, placement of a spatula horizontally between the lips may be introduced to improve awareness and build lip strength for the end goal of lip closure.

Homework

Carers and their children follow the individual guidelines given until the beginning of the EDS programme. Programmes may include activities for improvement of oral awareness, normalisation to touch, oral exploration and oral motor activities. Examples are contained in the homework handout (Form 4.11).

Sensory Groups
Jeni Malone

In children with EDS aversion, we need to consider the child's total sensory processing abilities, as it is possible that sensory issues may be involved either in the causation of, or contributing to the maintenance of EDS problems. Sensory processing is our link with the external environment from our internal environment. Where sensory defensiveness is seen it is usually in more than one sensory system (Kinnealy et al, 1995) and the child can put significant time and effort into the development of avoidance and coping measures, a trait often associated with children with EDS aversion.

All of the information we receive about the world comes to us through our sensory systems, for example the sense of touch, the sense of movement, the sense of body position and the sense of taste/smell. A difficulty taking in, processing or responding to this sensory information may mean that the child does not respond or responds in a way we do not expect. In pre-feeding work the aim is to:

1 Widen the child's sensory experiences in a safe, structured way to enable greater acceptance of a wider variety of textures and tastes.
2 Improve the child's ability to process this sensory information through:
   - Graded participation in a wide variety of sensory activities
   - Identification of the types of sensory activities that each individual child seeks out
   - Setting up a sensory diet/activity home programme for each child based on identified difficulties/needs
   - Supporting carers in participating in sensory activities with their child at a level which will enable achievement, and provide them with the skills to maintain, and alter when necessary, their child's sensory home programme.

The activity programme should include a range of activities aimed at appropriate levels for each individual child, to facilitate participation and to stimulate development of more effective processing of sensory information. The approach used here is not sensory integration as such but more like a 'sensory diet'-based strategy (Wilbarger, 1995; Wilbarger & Wilbarger, 2001). The aims of a sensory diet include reducing sensory defensiveness, promotion of optimal levels of arousal, and improvement of self regulation and bilateral organisation. Carers should be provided with a copy of the Sensory Group handout (Form 4.15), which can be found at the end of the chapter.

Sessions

While intervention is child-centred and process-orientated for the child, it is goal-orientated for the clinician. Goals for each session are set for each individual child, and communicated clearly to carers. Carers must facilitate the child in the group as an aid to carry-through of the programme at home. Depending on the structure of the course, carers will have participated in, or shortly will participate in, an education session in relation to sensory processing and setting up of their child's 'sensory diet'. This includes references for additional sensory activities (see Chapter 3).

Intervention will need to focus on proprioceptive/vestibular/tactile-based activities, preparing the whole nervous system for activities moving from hands to arms, face and into the mouth, thus helping to prepare the child for oral sensory and EDS sessions. Occupational therapists and speech & language therapists should liaise at this point in relation to a child's overall sensory processing, appropriate oral sensory activities and oral motor activities.

Two sensory group plans have been described below. These are ideas for activities and will need to be adapted to suit individual groups of children and available resources.

Parallel group
The first is a group plan (see Form 4.13) that uses six different areas in the room, each set up with an activity as listed in Table 28 (there are two multisensory areas). Each child works individually at a station with their carer to achieve their pre-determined goal, and then everyone moves on to the next station. It is important to have a quiet area in the room to facilitate any child who needs it. Three group plans are shown in Table 28 and can be repeated to provide six sessions. The child's participation in the group is recorded, as are specific goals for each child, and whether or not these were achieved. New goals are then set for the next group with the child's carer.

Two-part sensory group
The second sensory type group is in two parts:

1 An obstacle course to begin with, requiring the children to take turns and wait.
2 A tabletop activity with all the children around one table working on their own sensory goals.

Table 28: Parallel sensory group suggestions

Session	Activity
Parallel sensory session 1	Tactile/multisensory area
	Jumping in hoops
	Sitting on therapy ball (bouncing, holding rings on arms, throwing rings into container)
	Wheelbarrow walking
	Tactile/multisensory area
	Finger painting
	Choice activity
	Home books
Parallel sensory session 2	Tactile/multisensory area
	Stamping
	Prone on therapy ball (throwing beanbags at velcroed clown)
	Skittles
	Tactile/multisensory area
	Playdough (kneading in colours, cutting shapes)
	Choice activity
	Home books
Parallel sensory session 3	Sitting on therapy ball (bouncing, reaching down/forward/to side, placing rings on cones)
	Tactile/multisensory area
	Crawling through tunnel
	Scooter board (bringing beanbags to container)
	Tactile/multisensory area
	Lucky dip (in sand/rice/styrofoam)
	Choice activity
	Home books

This sensory group plan starts with a simple obstacle course that the children can move through in turn, progresses to a tactile-based activity and on to clear-up time signifying the end of the session. Participation and goals are recorded as for the previous group. Sample sensory group activity suggestions are listed in Table 29.

Table 29: Sample sensory group activity sessions

Day	Obstacle course	Table-top activity	End of session
Day 1	Basketball (use heavier ball) Each child jumps/steps into hoops Collects ball and carries back over head Take turns Replace ball by stepping into hoops	Playdough Choose colour and mix Roll into balls Flatten balls with hands Cut out shapes	Clear-up Wash-up Dry Rubbing cream
Day 2	Throw rings into container Each child crawls through tunnel Collects rings, one on each wrist, walks back with arms held out Throw rings into container Take turns to throw bags	Painting Finger painting Hand and face painting, each child picks design for face (carers instructed to use firm strokes towards mouth closure)	Clear-up Wash-up Dry Rubbing cream
Day 3	Skittles (use heavier balls) Each child stamps over to table (on feet shapes) Collect container with balls/skittles Take turns Step over rings coming back	Painting Blowing paint with straws Hand and face painting (carers encouraged to use firm strokes towards mouth closure)	Clear-up Wash-up Dry Rubbing cream

Homework

Each child will have a sensory diet set up in consultation with the clinician after assessment and this will continue to be the sensory home programme. The sensory groups should give the carers and children a chance to try out activities and ask questions, and empower them to integrate and implement the sensory diet in the home situation. The clinician must always be available to deal with queries or problems that arise. See Form 4.14 for sample Sensory Homework Sheet.

Daily Diary

The Daily Diary (Form 4.16) can be useful in helping carers evaluate the day's progress and plan the next day's goals. This helps both the clinicians in planning individualised goals and the carers in being actively involved in managing their own and their child's progress, and in unifying their thinking on all the day's activities.

Concluding the Fun before Food programme

The Feedback Form (Form 4.17), which carers fill in, helps the team to evaluate the Fun before Food programme. The carers and key-worker should meet to plan pre-feeding activities for the clients over the weeks between the pre-feeding and EDS elements of the programme. This time should be utilised as an opportunity to concentrate on developing those skills targeted by the clinicians in the various sessions and clearly outlined in the EDS books. Carers should be advised that progression to oral eating can be dependent on their application of these activities over this time.

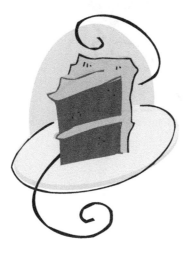

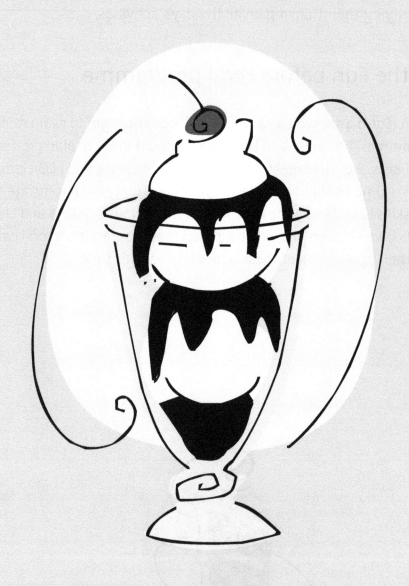

Chapter 4 Photocopiable master forms and sample forms

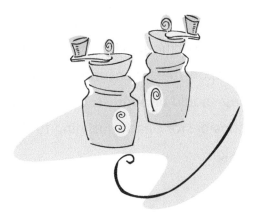

Form 4.1: Fun before Food Staff Guidelines

Please find enclosed the handouts included in the carer pack for your information. It is important that you both know and understand the aims and activities carried out in other sessions in order to:

- Effectively carry out your role as key-worker
- Gain a broad overview of the programme
- Fully integrate and align your specific goals with those of other team members and the overall programme goals.

Attendance

Your attendance at all sections of the course is not mandatory. However, you may want to participate actively in or observe sessions that are of interest to you. What is essential is that you gain as complete a picture as possible of the child and carer team for which you are key-worker. This may necessitate attendance at sessions for which you are not team leader. You should make yourself as available as possible for these reasons. You must always request the permission of the activity leader who is responsible for each session.

Activity leaders

- The activity leaders for each session/activity are agreed in advance and identified in the timetable. They are responsible for determining the goals and directing the activities of the sessions allocated to them.
- The activity leaders for each section will determine, in conjunction with the course co-ordinator, what staff are required to participate in their sessions. It is their responsibility to ensure they have enough staff in the room to facilitate activities. Any requests to participate in specific activities must go through activity leaders.
- The activity leader is also responsible for ensuring the timetable is adhered to. Any problems with timekeeping should be addressed to the course co-ordinator.
- The activity leader is responsible for clearly outlining to the carers what is expected from them within the session.

Page 1 of 3

Form 4.1: *continued*

■ The activity leader is responsible for ensuring that the individual is facilitated to meet the goals of the session/homework given, through individualising the programme where necessary, either directly or through the key-worker.

Key-workers

■ Key-workers are allocated before the programme begins.

■ The key-worker session provides carers and staff with an opportunity to meet together at the end of each day to resolve any outstanding issues, facilitate carry-over of recommendations and strategies, and revisit any areas which may need to be repeated for the benefit of either party.

■ Staff should be available to answer specific questions during sessions. Any other queries or clarifications should be kept for the key-worker session for whch there is a dedicated half-hour.

■ Please use this time with carers as effectively as possible.

■ The key-worker's role is to facilitate the carer's and child's progress and to co-ordinate with other staff members on their behalf if required.

■ Key-workers should consider participating in certain sessions to facilitate the child's and carer's progress – under the direction of the session leader.

Eating & Drinking & Swallowing books

■ Homework needs to be planned in advance.

■ All activity leaders should liaise with the activity leader for the EDS book session, so that this staff member knows what is required from each session in terms of homework.

Childminding

If staff do not require children to be present for any part of their sessions, they must arrange for the children to be looked after by liaising with the therapy assistants in advance.

Page 2 of 3

Form 4.1: *continued*

Clinical notes

A Case Note form should be filled out for each child after each session and filed in the tray.

Carers

The programme encourages active carer participation. Remember to:

- Praise carers even for small steps – build up confidence
- Model good practice
- Facilitate carers to carry out activities.

Room management

- Always tidy your treatment room after use
- Please clear away equipment
- Please wipe down surfaces
- Please brush floors.

Signed _____

Course co-ordinator

Form 4.2: Case Notes Master Form

Name of child

_____

Session title

_____

Date

_____

Day No. within programme

_____

Session goal

_____

Outcome

_____

Action/Plan

_____

Signed

_____

Title

_____

Once completed, this form is to be placed in this identified location _____

If you require a copy for your records please copy, but do not retain the original.

Form 4.3: Homework Handout

The aim of this part of Fun before Food is to review
and reinforce the day's activities
and
begin to work on homework that clinicians have
planned out after the sessions each day.

The clinicians feel that homework is an important
and fun part of the week as it helps to conclude each
of the day's events, and plan for carry-over onto the
rest of the day.

Form 4.4: Growing Big & Strong Handout

During the Fun before Food programme you and your child will be introduced to healthy eating in a fun way. Through stories and play activities you will learn about food and nutrition. The aims are:

To improve nutritional intake
To heighten awareness of food and its nutritional content
To introduce nutrient-dense foods
To broaden the range of food intake
To prepare for the Eating & Drinking & Swallowing programme

To eat healthily, children should choose from the four food groups:

Big & Strong Foods
Contain protein for growth and repair
eg Meat, Fish, Eggs, Beans, Peas and Lentils

Teeth & Bone Foods
Provide calcium for healthy bones and teeth
eg Milk, Cheese, Yoghurt

Energy Foods
Give you energy
eg Bread, Potatoes, Rice, Breakfast cereals, Pasta

Helping-hand Foods
Contain vitamins which are necessary for health
eg All fruit and vegetables (fresh, dried, tinned, frozen), fruit and vegetable juices.

Form 4.5: Normalisation Handout

Normalisation refers to activities to do with food that don't actually involve eating and drinking. The aims are:

- To provide experience of food in a non-threatening environment
- To provide you and your child with experience of food and food-related activities other than eating
- To extend your child's knowledge and sensory experience of food.

Session 1

A feely bag activity to explore food with the senses

Session 2

A pretend tea party using toys but real food

Session 3

We will visit a local supermarket. Each person will travel with their child in their own transport to:

NAME OF SHOP _____

ADDRESS _____

_____

DIRECTIONS _____

_____

Some shopping is included. We will provide you with the amount of _____;
you pay the extra if you go over budget!

Session 4

Cookery.

Form 4.6: Normalisation Homework Hints

- Use daily activities that involve food, from setting the table to washing up or loading the dishwasher.
- Shopping is a great activity as there is so much potential. Give children their own shopping list, which can include pictures of the food rather than words if this is developmentally more appropriate.
- Always comment or reference sensory aspects such as visual differences (eg in colour), temperature, smells, touch – whether in the supermarket or at home.
- Don't be afraid to mess! Children should be allowed to get dirty, mainly because this is how they learn about different foods, from feeling it on their hands to smelling it as it remains on their lips. Wiping is not encouraged during an activity and where possible children should clean themselves to give them further opportunities for sensory information. Wear aprons if you don't want clothing to get dirty, but be prepared for mess!

Instructions

- Choose to do two of the following activites and try to choose ones that you feel would be most useful to your child, not just those that are easiest to arrange!
- Complete the Eating & Drinking & Swallowing book with your child after you and they complete the activities.
- Encourage your child to show the book to another person and relate their achievements.

Activities

- Explore the kitchen together, look in food cupboards and the fridge, open jars and smell contents. If appropriate touch the food, also look at different utensils and tell your child about them, allow them to try using the utensils (eg mashing potatoes).
- Cook together: Make something for a family meal and then serve it. For example, Rice Krispie buns, Angel Delight, mousse, soup, a dip.
- Involve your child in routine tasks such as setting the table, clearing the table, washing up.
- Take your child shopping and repeat the shopping activities carried out during the group.

Page 1 of 2

Form 4.6: *continued*

EDS books

Using photos (especially for the shopping activity) or symbols for other activities, construct a record of what the child did using these visual representations and sentences such as:

Today I smelled _____ (eg a lemon)

It smelled _____ (eg funny, wicked, yummy)

Today I touched _____ (eg an apple, yoghurt)

It felt _____ (eg furry, like my teddy, smooth)

It was easy/difficult/fun/scary

We went shopping to _____ (paste in a photo)

We bought _____ (paste in package cover)

Form 4.7: Sample Food Play Chart

Name of child _____ Date _____

Completed by _____

Date	Food	Level	Response	Action
2/2/2006	Sweets, pasta shells	**D** medium coarseness	Horror initially, complied on modelling	Move to finer textures
	Lentils, maize	**D** finer textured	Tolerated well	Move to **WF**
3/2/2006	Bread dough	**WF**	Reluctantly tolerated, improved with time	Move to **WS**
	Treacle	**WS**	Tolerated well, licked finger	Try **WM**
4/2/2006	Yoghurt and sweets	**WM**	Total rejection Absolute aversion	Return to **WS**

Levels

D = Dry food play

WF = Wet firm consistency (dough)

WT = Wet tacky consistency (cooked pasta or rice)

WS = Wet semi-solid consistency (jelly)

WL = Wet liquid consistency (pouring custard or yoghurt)

WM = Wet mixed textures.

Form 4.8: Food Play Chart

Name of child _____ Date _____

Completed by _____

Date	Food	Level	Response	Action

Levels

P   = Pretend food play

D   = Dry food play

WF   = Wet firm consistency (dough)

WT   = Wet tacky consistency (cooked pasta or rice)

WS   = Wet semi-solid consistency (jelly)

WL   = Wet liquid consistency (pouring custard or yoghurt)

WM   = Wet mixed textures.

Form 4.9: Food Play Handout

The goal in the food play sessions is to introduce food as a fun and non-threatening activity.

Playing with food through structured activities will help to begin to desensitise your child to food that they see, hear, smell or touch.

Your child will become more confident when interacting with food, and it is hoped that this will help prepare him/her for oral eating.

The plan is to introduce pretend play followed by play with dry, wet and, finally, foods of mixed textures.

Form 4.10: Oral Motor Record Form

Name of child _____   Date _____

Session number _____

Oral facial awareness

Goal/s:

Achieved: yes/no

Details:

Next step:

Normalisation to touch

Goal/s:

Achieved: yes/no

Details:

Next step:

Oral imitation

Goal/s:

Achieved: yes/no

Details:

Next step:

Oral motor activities

Goal/s:

Achieved: yes/no

Details:

Next step:

Signed _____   Position _____

Form 4.11: Oral Motor Homework Example Handout

Oral awareness

Look at different parts of the face and mouth. Touch each part as you name them. Find different parts on your face as well as on your child's. Explore different facial movements. For example:

- Lips: 'Find your lips', 'Let's blow a kiss', 'Can you smile?', 'We can open and close our lips'.
- Biting: Talk about how we can bite – we open and close our jaw.
- Drinking: Talk about drinking and how we move the different parts of our mouth when we drink. Let your child watch himself in the mirror while he sips from a straw. Make him aware of the lips and how they close around the straw.

Normalisation to touch

Use your hands and apply firm pressure touch. Begin near the temporo-mandibular joint and move towards the lips. Use firm presses. Apply firm presses with the index finger around your child's lips. Start near the corner of the lip and move to the middle. First above the top lip and then below the bottom lip. Use different textures on your child's face. Describe the textures to him. Sing songs and play 'patty-cake' on his cheeks as you bounce him on your knee.

Work on the concepts wet and dry. Explore these language concepts in games and activities with all the parts of the body, for example during bath time talk about how our bodies are wet and how we now have to dry them. Discover those things that can make our face wet and dry, for example when cleaning our face or brushing our teeth.

Oral exploration

Use oral toys to help your child explore. Let him hold a toy and put it to his lips. Describe what is happening. Talk about the textures of the different items. Introduce the Chewy Tube again. First let the child hold it and then encourage him to put it inside his mouth. Experiment with biting.

Page 1 of 2

Form 4.11: *continued*

Oral motor exercises

- Bubbles – Catch a bubble on the wand – use your fingers on the child's cheeks to gently pull his lips forward to assist with lip rounding. Attempt to use the bubble face to help with lip rounding.
- Whistle/horn – Make your child aware of his lips as he puts the horn inside his mouth. Encourage your child to see how many times he can blow the horn. Talk about blowing 'Ready steady BLOW'.
- Straws – Let your child use his special straw for drinking – this is an excellent exercise to help tongue retraction.
- Mouth rhymes – Use these to practise different movements of the lips/jaw/face.

Form 4.12: Oral Motor Skills Handout

Aims

1 To develop oral facial awareness through:
   - Knowledge of the different parts of the face and mouth, and their functions
   - Working towards accepting touch in and around the mouth.
2 To increase your child's confidence in exploring oral motor movements.
3 To develop oral motor skills.

Session plans

In the three sessions, different parts of the face and mouth will be targeted. Fun activities will be introduced to help your child understand the process of eating and to practise the different movements we need in order to chew, lick, bite and suck.

Session 1: My face and mouth

This is an introduction to the different parts of the face and mouth. We use mirror work to look for and identify different parts of our face. We talk about each part and we practise different movements of each part, such as facial expressions, biting, blowing a kiss, opening and closing mouth etc.

Session 2: All the things I can do with my mouth

We explore the mouth and its movements in this session with the use of non-food items. We look at movements of the lips, teeth and tongue, and practise biting, blowing and licking during fun oral exploration activities.

Session 3: Exercises just for me!

In this session, children will partake in activities devised to meet their specific needs. Exercises will be demonstrated to you so that you can follow these guidelines at home.

Form 4.13: Parallel Sensory Group Form

Name of child _____

Session 1		Activity	Comments
	1	Tactile/multisensory area	
	2	Jumping in hoops	
	3	Sitting on therapy ball	
		Bouncing	
		Holding rings on arms	
		Throwing rings into	
		container	
	4	Wheelbarrow walking	
	5	Tactile/multisensory area	
	6	Finger painting	
	7	Choice activity	
	8	Home books	
Session 2		**Activity**	**Comments**
	1	Tactile/multisensory area	
	2	Stamping	
	3	Prone on therapy ball	Note: use large wooden clown with
		Throwing beanbags	Velcro to catch beanbags
		at clown	
	4	Skittles	
	5	Tactile/multisensory area	
	6	Playdough	
		Kneading in colours	
		Cutting shapes	
	7	Choice activity	
	8	Home books	

Form 4.13: *continued*

Session 3		Activity	Comments
	1	Tactile/multisensory area	
	2	Crawling through tunnel	
	3	Sitting on therapy ball 　Bouncing 　Reaching down/ 　forward/to side 　Placing rings on cones	
	4	Scooter board 　Bringing beanbags to 　container	
	5	Tactile/multisensory area	
	6	Lucky dip 　In sand/rice/styrofoam	
	7	Choice activity	
	8	Home books	

Page 2 of 2

Form 4.14: Sample Sensory Homework Sheet

1 Never force your child to complete a task he does not seem ready for.

2 Give consistent reinforcement for completed tasks; do not reprimand non-completed tasks.

3 Activities incorporating proprioceptive and vestibular information:
   ■ Heavy marching, jumping, wheelbarrow walk, seat walking (while sitting on floor with legs straight, that is, using arms to lift and push body), tug-of-war, foot-to foot cycling with friend
   ■ Carrying heavy objects such as books, helping move furniture, chairs etc
   ■ Roll up in blanket, duvet, towel (make hot dog or sandwich). Wrap tightly in bath towel after bath (with firm hugs)
   ■ Firm rubdown with towel before and after bath
   ■ Rub in lotion firmly – into hands and face if allowed. Let your child start this, rub into whole body after bath
   ■ Deep touch pressure to limbs/torso, body hugs, hand squeezes.

4 Continue to give opportunities to partake in a wide variety of tactile tasks, beginning with activities as above, choosing short tasks and taking frequent breaks, and include tasks such as:
   ■ Playdough – including mixing and stirring ingredients, rolling dough, pounding/banging dough, pinching dough, kneading in colours
   ■ Lucky dip – searching for hidden toys/objects in a variety of materials such as sand, pasta, rice, dried peas, styrofoam packaging, small squares/pieces of newspaper (get your child to tear these up), or use any other paper, water, soil (if working in garden with hidden bulbs for planting). Look at what you have to hand and use these items
   ■ Painting – finger painting, pressing fingers/hands into paint. Fill in outline with dots (fingertips)
   ■ Experiment with a variety of washcloths, sponges, bath-mitts – allowing your child to do this him or herself.

5 Oral stimulation
   ■ Provide deep pressure to hands, arms and up to face and mouth before meals.
   ■ Intraoral stimulation (to liaise with speech & language therapist for programme).

Form 4.15: Sensory Group Handout

All of the information we receive about the world comes to us through our sensory systems, for example:

- The sense of touch
- The sense of movement
- The sense of body position
- The sense of taste/smell.

A difficulty taking in, processing or responding to this sensory information may mean that your child does not respond, or responds in a way we do not expect.

In the sensory groups the aim is to:

- Broaden your child's sensory experiences in a safe, structured way to enable greater acceptance of a wider variety of textures and tastes
- Improve your child's ability to process this sensory information through:
  - Graded participation in a wide variety of sensory activities
  - Identification of the types of sensory activities that each individual child seeks out
  - Setting up a sensory diet/activity home programme for each child, based on identified difficulties/needs.

Form 4.16: Fun before Food Daily Diary Form

Please fill in this sheet at the end of each day and return to the course co-ordinator the following morning.

Name of child _____

Date _____   Day   1   2   3

This is what my/our child did today that was a step towards better eating and drinking skills:

_____

_____

_____

This is what I/we learned today that might help my/our child with eating and drinking:

_____

_____

_____

_____

This is what I/we think is required for my/our child tomorrow:

_____

_____

_____

This is what I/we think is required for me/us tomorrow:

_____

_____

_____

Signed _____

Name/s _____

Form 4.17: Fun before Food Programme Feedback Form

Date _____

Please fill in the Feedback form so we can adapt and improve the course in future. Your input and advice is much appreciated in making the programme better for carers, staff and children. Thank you for helping.

Please rate on a 1–5 scale where 1 = very poor, 2 = poor, 3 = okay/average,

4 = good, 5 = excellent

Activity	Rating	Comments
Sensory group		
Oral motor		
Food play		
Normalisation		
Key-worker meetings		

Eating & Drinking & Swallowing books:

_____

Other comments:

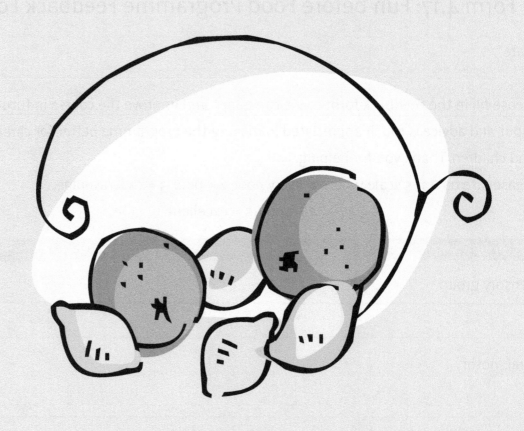

Chapter 5

Stage 4

Fun with Food:
The Eating & Drinking &
Swallowing (EDS) programme

The aim of the EDS programme is to provide multiple opportunities for carers *and* children to practise and develop new skills in a highly supportive environment. The child is given repeated opportunities to achieve EDS goals as set by carers (with guidance from clinicians), and carers have multiple opportunities to develop goal-setting and management skills. Although the overall aim of the programme is to develop oral EDS skills and oral intake, it is also an effective means of getting both carers and children motivated to start working on ways of overcoming EDS difficulties, and provide them with the confidence to continue progress outside the clinical context.

Therefore the core of the EDS section is:
1 Repeated EDS opportunities
2 Carer support
3 Goal-setting skill development
4 Carer–child interaction/behaviour management.

What is required?

Requirements for the EDS element of the Fun with Food programme are listed in Table 30.

Remember that carers eat with their children and will also require lunch and so on. Quantities must reflect this.

Weekend break

The EDS programme is typically run with a two-day break in the middle (usually a Saturday and Sunday) to:

■ Give carers a chance to carry over development of EDS skills and management strategies in the home environment, but with the opportunity of coming back to continue with the programme under the guidance of clinicians
■ Iron out any problems which may have arisen during the break.

Table 30: Requirements for EDS elements of the programme

Item	Details
Accommodation	• A big group dining room with separate tables and chairs for each child and carer team. Tables and chairs should be child-sized • A child chill-out room set up with child-friendly activities, eg videos, drawing corner, train corner, dress-up area, sand play etc • A carer chill-out room for discussing and analysing performance after eating and drinking activities, and for carer support groups • A kitchen or kitchen area for selecting and preparing dishes with microwave, kettle, toaster and dishwasher or sink
Utensils	Plates big and small, cups, glasses, cutlery and a range of adapted utensils and cutlery
Food	A selection of food covering the range of consistencies and tastes, for example: A range of jar baby foods reflecting both sweet and savoury tastes and varying textures Juices, water, milk Cartons of custard, creamed rice, yoghurts, ice-cream Mash (potato) Beans, spaghetti (tins), mini-pizzas, breads Protein foods such as ham and cheese Biscuits, crisps, sweets Spices, various sauces, ketchup Order in foods such as chips, sausages etc. These are also available in freezer packs or come partly cooked.

Opening progress evaluations

Each day can be started with progress evaluations or a nutritional session with the aim of providing an impetus to the day's activities. In evaluating progress, carers are required to appraise homework and the previous evening's EDS activities and provide feedback to the group on:

1 Their evaluation of how their child performed
2 Their evaluation of how they performed
3 One positive and one negative outcome
4 Reasons for success and failure.

Other carers are encouraged to comment and support. This focus on continuing in-depth analysis of performance and outcomes facilitates appropriate goal setting by carers, in addition to helping them develop self-reliance in interpreting successes and failures along the road to oral eating.

Early morning nutrition session
Marie Kennedy

First day lecture
On the first day of the EDS programme, the dietitian hosts a 'Go for it!' lecture. The aim of this lecture is to provide the impetus for, and confidence to pursue, EDS goals, particularly for the carers of the tube feeders, and those who are concerned that their child might lose weight. The carers are provided with the knowledge to facilitate moving forward. Information given is based both on general nutrition knowledge required and the dietitian's evaluations of the children. Any recommendations such as for reducing or changing tube-feed volumes should be made by the qualified dietitian on the team and always in the context of the individual's needs. Depending on the child or children involved, carers may also benefit from the presence of a medical consultant to allay fears and provide guidelines.

Areas to focus on include those outlined in Table 31.

Monitoring nutrition

At the start of each day the dietitian meets with the child and carer.

- The child is weighed and recorded
- The progress of each child and tolerance of any sip supplement is discussed
- Recommendations may be made for trial of supplements and volume changes
- A record of any significant volume of food and drink is taken
- The carers and dietitian set nutritional targets
- Hydration is monitored. Any water, milk or fruit juice taken is recorded
- If tube-feeding is still being used it may be reduced to facilitate oral EDS development
- It is ensured that daily dietary intake meets nutritional requirements for children.

Table 31: Go for it! themes

Area of focus	Description
Individual nutrition issues	Discuss nutritional issues of the individuals, in particular in the Fun with Food course, as relevant
Medical & Nutritional stability	Children are stable medically and nutritionally (pre-requisite for the course). For example: The children are healthy; there are no extra demands for energy, protein, vitamins and minerals. The children do not have high temperature, vomiting, diarrhoea, infections, burns, wounds, fractures, and are not recovering from surgery
Nourishment	The children are well nourished, both oral and tube feeders. Tube feeders have been consistently receiving adequate nutrition for age and height over a long period of time through their feeding tubes. For example: Iron – they are not anaemic and have good iron stores Calcium – they have a good supply for healthy bones and teeth and also have good stores of calcium Energy and protein and vitamins A, B, C and D. Intakes are adequate to meet recommended dietary guidelines for age and height
Tube-feed reductions	Make recommendations for tube-feed reductions, such as tube-feed reduced by 50%. The remainder of tube-feed will continue to supply energy, protein, vitamins, minerals and fluids. Each child must have 500ml of fluid/feed daily via tube. Don't forget that the tube is there to top up fluids very quickly – if necessary A further tube-feed reduction of 100ml each night during the five-day programme to initiate a sense of hunger and thirst. (*These are generic guidelines only and any changes to tube-feed intake should be made by a qualified dietitian, based on the child's individual needs*)
Use of oral supplements	Why they might be used

continued →

Table 31: *continued*

Area of focus	Description

Hydration	Reiterate importance of fluid intake for both tube and oral eaters. Discuss fluid intake especially:
	    Overfilling with fluids
	    Fluids and appetite suppression
	    Necessity for children to receive sufficient but not excessive fluids daily
	 It is safe to proceed if there has not been a recent rapid fluid loss (eg vomiting, diarrhoea), or the child has not been chronically dehydrated
	 Revisit Signs of Dehydration (see Chapter 3)

Weight loss	Discuss possible weight loss Discuss nutritional stability of all children prior to programme and constant weight monitoring by dietitian which facilitates confidence in moving forward with oral goals.

Mid-programme break tasks

Mid-programme break (eg weekend) tasks are set, for example:

■ Tube feeds to be further reduced by 100ml each night over the two-day break
■ For non-tube feeders try: two new foods, eg chicken (four pieces), apple (bite)
■ Structure meal times, eg breakfast, lunch, dinner.

Eating & Drinking & Swallowing activities

Videotaping

Prior to videotaping a handout is given to carers explaining the 'How to' of videotaping (Form 5.1). Videotaping, as discussed in Chapter 2, is an integral part of the approach to development of EDS skills. Carers are required to evaluate both their own and their child's performance in order to facilitate further progress and development of goal-setting skills. The clinician facilitating this attempts to be as non-directive as possible, but may need to develop a carer's thinking around performance or forward planning. The use of open questions can help with this. In addition, this is an opportunity to praise, encourage and reinforce both the child and carer's performances.

Organising EDS activities

Sometimes it is better to have a theme (breakfast, dessert, lunch etc) to sessions to help with the organisation of foodstuffs and general goal-setting skills. However, with some children it is essential to stick to the same goals or graded developments of them at each subsequent session. The choice lies with the clinicians and carers and is based on the individual child's needs and progress. Clinicians should always set sessions up so that carers have an opportunity to 'eat' or model eating & drinking & swallowing.

The clinician can plan the day, therefore, using either of the two options below: the meals approach or the developmental approach.

Meals approach
The meals approach facilitates the use of a range of foods and reflects more closely the mealtime structures utilised in the home environment. It can also encourage carers to attempt a range of goals, that is, to not play safe. An example is given in Table 32.

Developmental approach
In the developmental approach the individual goals are clearly based on the child's and carer's performance on the previous meals. It reflects clearly an individualised, graded, step-by-step approach to developing EDS skills. Carers base their next goal for the next activity on performance in the last activity. The best approach is what suits the individual at that time.

Goal setting for EDS activities

Children with oral eating aversion (with and without sensory issues) both have a genuine fear of new foods, and put a lot of effort into avoidance strategies and coping measures,

Table 32: Sample EDS activity organisation

EDS Activity	Structure
EDS activity 1	Breakfast
EDS activity 2	Snack
EDS activity 3	Lunch
EDS activity 4	Dessert
EDS activity 5	Snack

hence the need to apply a consistent, goal-directed approach. Goal setting is the most important part of the EDS programme (Form 5.2 can be given to carers to remind them what they need to consider in setting goals), and requires a significant amount of time during the day, before, during and after the EDS activity itself, as shown below.

A pre-EDS goal-setting session to decide the goals
The goal form (Form 5.3 or 5.4) should be used for the purpose of deciding the goals. Writing down goals is important – they should not just be verbalised, and carers should have their goals clear in their mind before commencing the activity.

The actual EDS activity
Carrying out EDS goals.

Post-EDS session
Time is needed after the EDS activity to analyse child and carer performance, and whether the goals worked. If yes, why? If no, why not? Were the goals inappropriate? Did the carer change the goals? Start pleading or negotiating?

The importance of this analysis component cannot be understated. It gives carers the time they need to review, and to forward plan. Encourage carers to take their goal form and mark it using the scale outlined on the forms. Clinicians should also do the same, to provide a balance to carer ratings. In our experience, carers' ratings of their child typically start by undervaluing the achievements of the child, however small. Any contradiction in ratings should be discussed. During post-EDS activity review, carers are reminded, where necessary, of the main principles of goal setting, most specifically:

> **Take small steps**
> **Be specific – use measurable outcomes**
> **Plan your language**
> **Plan the reinforcement**

These may need to be reiterated at each post-EDS review until the carers have had repeated, or enough, practice setting goals. In addition, the carers' and children's performance may give rise to specific suggestions. Always try to make this as carer-led as possible, for example, 'What do you think went wrong?' or 'What behaviour could you change next time to facilitate goal achievement?'

Sometimes, however, carers are so caught up in the emotions of EDS, in particular with feelings of failure, that they require direction and guidance. In such circumstances the clinician may decide to direct the carer in order to facilitate progress. For example, some carers start by setting goals for eating of complete meals for children who take nothing orally. Guidance will be necessary in these cases in order to ensure more appropriate and achievable goals. Small graded steps are essential to ensuring success: too big a step is a recipe for failure.

General reminders can be useful and are sometimes best written so that carers can see them in the carer room, for example on a flip chart/notice board. They should be individualised based on Assessment Day performance, and added to as issues arise on an ongoing basis but can include:

> **No pleading**
> **No negotiation**
> **Don't be tempted to change the rules when on a roll**
> **Be neutral – your emotions should not be obvious in your face, voice or language**
> **Do keep your focus**
> **Do have realistic goals**
> **Take small steps**
> **Encourage independence**

Setting up EDS activities

After the goals have been set for each particular EDS activity, the carers are required to set up EDS activities as outlined below. Carers, and not clinicians, carry out these activities to ensure more successful carry-over in the long term.

- Prepare the room – are there chairs and a table suitable for the child and carer?
- Table preparation – are utensils and, for example, placemats laid out? Placemats can be individualised to help the child settle and adapt (use photos and a laminator).
- Each child should be encouraged to be involved in the preparation for an EDS activity. Use plastic storage boxes with their utensils, equipment, special food, placements, and so on inside. Children can bring these to the table and assist in setting up. It helps them mentally prepare for the EDS activity.
- Food preparation – have the food ready to go, based on the goal.
- Clothing preparation – is the child in old clothes or has he a bib, if appropriate to developmental level, physical skills or behaviour?

- Self-preparation – review agreed goals.
- Re-advise the carer to become neutral both behaviourally and facially.

Carer support group

Within the EDS element of the programme, time is given to carers to facilitate peer support, positive thinking and resolution of any issues relevant for them in implementing the programme. This is essential, as change can be hard to accept and implement and EDS difficulties are not always understood by other people, be they family or friends. The carer support group gives carers an opportunity to:

1 Meet with other carers
2 Share information
3 Benefit from the group support
4 Have time out in a hectic and somewhat difficult week
5 Develop their own awareness of issues
6 Provide peer support.

In addition, as the demand on carers (and children) for behaviour and attitude changes grow, the carer support group can:

1 Help considerably by facilitating this change through discussion and peer support.
2 Help carers understand their own, and other carers' issues, building on that 'I'm not alone' feeling in addition to building confidence in their abilities.

Activity suggestions

Sessions have no set agenda and are typically carer-led and facilitated by an experienced counsellor such as a psychologist or social worker. This is not mandatory, however, as many therapists are skilled at leading carer groups.

Discussions can be initiated using the following topics:

1 Family feeding problems
2 Child's EDS problems
3 Coping skills and strategies
4 Having a child with a disability

5 Nurturing/self-care
6 Attitudes to food and eating.

The Carer Support Group Handout (Form 5.5) is useful for explaining to carers the purpose of the group, and can be added to the carer pack.

Concurrent child session

The child session runs concurrently with the carer support group and can be directed by the individual child's needs and the resources available to the team. Examples of ways to use this session are given below.

Activity suggestions

- If there are sufficient staff available, individual sessions along the lines of the pre-feeding activities (eg an oral motor activity for one child, a sensory processing session for another) can be organised.
- A group session similar to any in the Fun before Food programme element.
- A time-out/chill-out session away from the intensity of the programme, and conducted through active play, can be beneficial. Always follow this with quiet play – calming down before the next EDS activity. Active play activities can be gym-based activities, playground time and indoor games such as musical chairs.
- Low-level stimulation or quiet play can vary from nap time, to low-key child videos or DVDs. The focus should be on quietness and calming down.
- Positive imagery, communication and commentary about food can be reinforced, for example, through food songs/nursery rhymes, food stories/books.
- A child-centred 'Food makes me feel …' session.
  This session can also be held during the Fun before Food programme. The clinician can bring to the session:
  (a) Different faces representing different emotions. These should be enlarged to highlight the emotion involved. Examples are: sad, mad, happy, afraid. Labels used should be simple.
  (b) Pictures of food, preferably as realistic as possible, for example cut-out pictures from magazines, or actual foods/empty cartons. There should be representations of the various food groups, that is, 'child' foods, 'junk' foods, textured foods and foods that are known to be preferred and non-preferred based on the child's Tastes & Textures Questionnaire.

(c) A Velcro board or big cardboard board and various fittings by which each child can physically attach the aforementioned emotion pictures to the wall. The wall of a room can also be used (or corridor if space is limited).

The aim is to encourage children to express their emotions around various foods – without judgement. This should be a fun and expressive session and is particularly suitable for children who are verbal, although non-verbal children can join in the fun and should also benefit from it. A consistent phrase should be used that the children can then learn to utilise in concrete communications with their carers as they progress in their understanding of themselves and eating. For example:

> '(Identify item)   makes me feel   (Identify emotion) '

eg   'Beans   make me feel   sick!'

The clinicians in the group should join in to normalise positive and negative responses to food.

Wrap Up: framing progress

The Wrap Up session is the penultimate activity of the day. The aim is to:

- Provide daily feedback and analysis
- Keep carers on track
- Pull together all information learned during the day
- Identify homework
- Prevent overload/confusion occurring.

Activity suggestions

1 The group should discuss the day's activities, carers should analyse outcomes and performance and the clinician should establish reasons for interpretations. For example, if a carer goal has been met but the carer remains unhappy because the child still isn't eating full oral intake, this needs to be discussed in the context of overnight cures, child achievements, and carer expectations – both immediate and long term. Constant challenging means carers will be more realistic both within and after the programme. Failure to facilitate carer analysis in this way could result in long-term failure of oral eating goals.

   The use of simple statistics also helps in the analysis of skills. For example, provide carers with the percentage of meals for which their targets have been met. If goals are not successful, the reasons for this, including the possibility of unrealistic goals, should be probed. Forms 5.6 (Daily Evaluation Form) and 5.7 (Fun with Food Daily Diary) can facilitate this activity. The Daily Diary (as for the Fun before Food element of the programme) can be useful in helping carers evaluate the day's progress and plan the next day's goals during the evening. This assists both clinicians in planning individualised goals and carers in being actively involved in managing their own and their child's progress, and in unifying their thinking on all the day's activities.

2 Agree homework, both nutritional and EDS: give a written outline.
3 Identify any outstanding concerns.

Homework planning/Key-worker meeting

The homework planning/key-worker meeting aims to facilitate carry-over of EDS goals into the home environment for the remainder of the day. The programme day typically finishes in the early afternoon – the intensity of the programme means it may be unwise to continue beyond this point. However, some carers and children may benefit from a further EDS activity to end the day, and this can be negotiated/discussed between clinician and carers.

The key-worker should meet with the carer to:

1 Review and reinforce the day's activities and child's and carer's progress
2 Plan evening EDS goals.

Eating & Drinking & Swallowing books (as per Fun before Food) can be used, with the focus this time on actual eating & drinking & swallowing (eg using pictures). Sentences such as those listed in Table 33 can be constructed:

Reviewing aims

At the end of the EDS programme (and More Food Review Days), carers and clinicians together should review aims made at the start of the course and during the particular section of the programme, and write aims for the period between sections of the programme (eg between More Food Review Days). The latter is most important, because it is essential for both carers and clinicians to keep goals on track, and it facilitates longer-term planning for carers. These aims are different from EDS goal setting, in that they are broader; they represent a longer period of time and therefore more general goals.

Table 33: EDS book example

Action	Body part (with my)	Amount	Food item (paste in picture)
Today I			
Smelled	Nose	A little bit	Juice
Touched	Hands	One	Crisp
Tasted/licked	Lips	A cup	Beans
Bit	Teeth	Corner	Bread
Chewed	Mouth/Tongue	Three	Chips
Swallowed	Throat	A small spoon	Yoghurt

The final review day in particular should revisit initial programme aims made during the Food for Thought carer programme so that carers can both chart progress and review the realism of aims. Form 5.8 is useful for this activity, and copies should be kept in individual files to facilitate review.

The team can also encourage carers to rate aims – both their own and the team's – using Form 5.9. This provides another opportunity to evaluate progress, appropriateness of aims and facilitate forward planning.

Sample aims are given in Table 34.

Table 34: Sample aims

Carer's aims
Try mashed and wet mixed textures
Develop independent feeding
Increase water intake
Trial spicy tastes
Try new spoon

Clinician's aims
Keep on two tube feeds daily as prescribed
Focus on independent feeding
Continue on purée consistencies

Upwards and Onwards session

The Upwards and Onwards session occurs on the last day of the EDS programme and its overall aim is to motivate carers to continue with the programme. It helps to:

1 Revise the programme
2 Review the performance of carers and children
3 Identify potential pitfalls
4 Provide motivation for continuation of programme guidelines
5 Address any outstanding concerns
6 Reinforce progress made.

Activity suggestions

- Brainstorm how the course went and why
- Key-worker and carers to analyse development in all targeted areas
- Brainstorm potential pitfalls
- Review carer goals and discuss whether they were realistic
- Identify carer needs at end of course and respond accordingly
- Reinforce positive developments
- Give general advice such as:
  - Monitor weight gain first then address the EDS problem
  - Make short- and long-term EDS and nutritional goals
  - Have realistic expectations – allow time to achieve goals
  - Have regular mealtimes
  - When introducing new foods, ideally eat with the child. Imitation of peers and adults is a powerful tool to encourage children to try new food.
- Fill out EDS Programme Evaluation Form (Form 5.10).

Chapter 5 Photocopiable master forms and sample forms

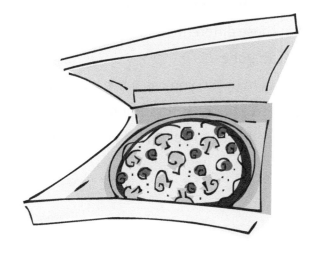

Form 5.1: Videotaping Handout for Carer

Videotaping is a standard part of the course and you and your child will be repeatedly taped, both for a record of your child's EDS skills and for therapeutic purposes. Tapes are not used for other activities outside this programme unless you specifically permit it. You are entitled to take a copy of the tape with you at the end of the programme – just let us know if you require a copy. And please don't worry about 'acting' or how you look on video etc. We know it's easier said than done - but you will get used to it!

Remember:

1   You are required to be as natural as possible! The video needs to be as accurate a representation of 'normal' as possible. Do not encourage your child, either in advance or on the day, to be on his 'best behaviour' because of the video – we need to see what really happens. Treat his behaviour as you would if you were at home. Use the same language, same reactions and so on.

2   Do not use statements such as 'Eat for the lady', 'The lady wants to see if you will eat for mummy' etc.

3   You are required to give your child preferred and non-preferred food and drink items. Preferred items are those which he will take relatively willingly; if he has none – don't worry – this is okay. Non-preferred food items are those which your child typically refuses when you offer them. It will be informative for the therapists to see how your child copes in these different situations. Please attempt at least one food and drink item in both categories.

4   The video will last up to 15 minutes; you can leave before then if you are finished. Your child is not required to eat a specific amount – remember, the point of the video is not to feed your child but to get an idea of how your child behaves at eating time.

Form 5.2: Overall Goal-Setting Guidelines

Before eating:

Identify goal (goals)

Identify reinforcement

Identify language (keywords)

Form 5.3: EDS Goal Form 1

Name of child _____ Date _____

Day No: 1   2   3   4   5   *(circle)*

Eating & Drinking & Swallowing Activity No _____

Identify goals:

1 _____

_____

2 _____

_____

3 _____

_____

Identify keywords/sentences to be used:

_____

_____

_____

_____

Identify reinforcement:

_____

_____

_____

Analyse how child did:

	Carer rating	Therapist rating
Goal 1:	_____	_____
Goal 2:	_____	_____
Goal 3:	_____	_____

Rate from 1 to 5 where: 1 is very poor/not achieved at all, and: 5 is excellent/achieved

Please return to Course co-ordinator

Form 5.4: EDS Goal Form 2

Name of child _____ Date _____

Day No: 1   2   3   4   5   *(circle)*

Eating & Drinking & Swallowing activity: Breakfast
Goal _____
Keywords _____
Reinforcement _____

Eating & Drinking & Swallowing activity: Snack
Goal _____
Keywords _____
Reinforcement _____

Eating & Drinking & Swallowing activity: Lunch
Goal _____
Keywords _____
Reinforcement _____

Eating & Drinking & Swallowing activity: Dessert/post-lunch
Goal _____
Keywords _____
Reinforcement _____

Eating & Drinking & Swallowing activity: Homework
Goal _____
Keywords _____
Reinforcement _____

Form 5.5: Carer Support Group Handout

Dear Carer

We recognise that eating, drinking & swallowing difficulties are not always understood by family and friends and can be difficult to manage on a day-to-day basis. Throughout the Fun with Food programme we would like to offer you an opportunity to meet with other carers. The purpose of this group will be to share information and to benefit from group support.

You can see from your timetable when these groups will run. This is set aside as time out for you.

I would also like to meet with you once on an individual basis at some time during the programme. However, this is at your discretion.

My phone number is _____

Looking forward to working with you.

Signed _____
     Counsellor

Form 5.6: Daily Evaluation Form

Name of child _____ Date _____

% of intake today – tube vs oral

Tube _____%   Oral _____%

Is this progress?   Yes _____   No _____

How many bites/spoonfuls did child take at the end of today vs yesterday?

Number yesterday _____   Number today _____

Tick the place of contact for today

Touch/hands _____   Smell/nose _____

Taste/lips _____   Swallow/mouth _____

% of meals today for which goals were met?

20% _____   40% _____   60% _____   80% _____   100% _____

What one thing did your child do today that was progress?

_____

_____

What one thing did you do today that you feel was evidence of progress?

_____

_____

Form 5.7: Fun with Food Daily Diary

Please fill in this sheet after each day and return to the course co-ordinator the following morning.

Name of child _____

Date _____ Day   1   2   3   *(circle)*

This is what my/our child did today that was a step towards better eating & drinking skills:

_____
_____
_____

This is what I/we learned today that may help my/our child with eating and drinking:

_____
_____
_____

This is what I/we think is required for my/our child tomorrow:

_____
_____
_____

This is what I/we think is required for me/us tomorrow:

_____
_____
_____

Signed _____

Form 5.8: Intervening Aims Form

Fun with Food

Eating & Drinking & Swallowing programme

Intervening Aims Form

Goals from end of _____ *to* _____

Child's name _____

Clinical staff	Carer
1	1
2	2
3	3
4	4
5	5
6	6
Identify priority aim:	Identify priority aim:

Form 5.9: Aims Rating Form

Rate the aims from:

EDS programme ☐

Review Day 1 ☐

Review Day 2 ☐

Review Day 3 ☐

Review Day 4 ☐

How well did we all succeed with regard to your aims/the clinician's aims? Please rate them from 1–5 where:

1 = did not meet the aim at all, 0% of the aim

2 = made a small amount of progress, maybe 25%

3 = made some progress, maybe 50%

4 = made lots of progress, perhaps 75%

5 = made excellent progress, 100% progress

Rate each aim individually and then give an overall score for overall progress. Both carers and staff will be rating their own and each other's aims during this session.

Form 5.9: *continued*

Name of child _____ Date _____

Carer's aims	Rating

Professional's aims	Rating

Overall progress comments	

Page 2 of 2

Form 5.10: EDS Programme Evaluation Form

Please fill in the feedback form so we can adapt and improve the course in future. Your input and advice is much appreciated in making the programme better for carers, staff and children. Thank you for helping.

Please rate on a 1–5 scale where 1 = very poor, 2 = poor, 3 = okay/average,

4 = good, 5 = excellent

Activity	Rating	Comments
Progress evaluations – early morning session		
Weigh in		
EDS sessions		
Wrap up		
Carer support group		
Key-worker meetings		

Other comments:

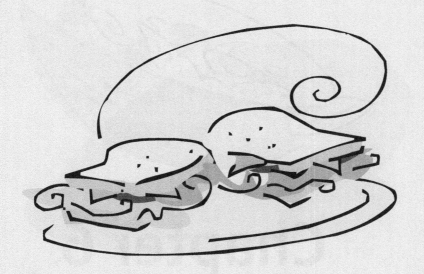

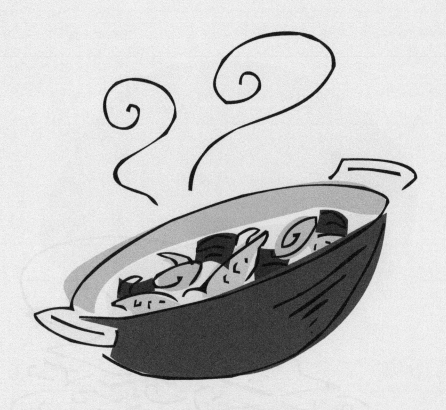

Chapter 6

STAGE 5

More Food Review Days

> **The aim of Review Days is threefold:**
> - **To monitor progress**
> - **To provide ongoing support and education**
> - **To facilitate further development of eating & drinking & swallowing (EDS) skills.**

Review Days can be held at whatever intervals clinicians and carers deem appropriate. However, it is recommended that a Review Day is held within one month of the course to ensure fairly immediate support for development. Review days can be run at either one or three monthly intervals thereafter, up to around the one year point. Discretion should then be used to decide if it is appropriate to continue with them. It can be beneficial to run joint days of various groups, perhaps once a year, to provide closure and hand-over to carers.

Activity suggestions

More Food Review Day timetable samples are shown in Appendix 1. Content typically consists of the following:

1 Review of previous aims and performance, and setting of new aims for the day (see previous chapters). Form 6.1 can be used for this purpose.
2 Rate goals from EDS course/previous Review Days.
3 Outline encouraging and discouraging developments (Form 6.3).
4 Reassessment (see Chapter 2 for forms).
5 EDS activities (see Chapter 5 for forms and activities).
6 Carer support group (see Chapter 5).
7 Nutritional redirection.
8 Evaluation of progress blockers. It can be worthwhile to probe for factors that may be negatively impacting on progress (Form 6.2).
9 Carers can find it useful to receive concrete feedback about their child's progress. Ways to do this include:
   - Use statistics. This can also provide carers with concrete evidence from which to interpret progress (see Form 6.4)
   - Other carers to comments on child's progress. Use of starter phrases such as 'What I remember about *(name's)* first day of the course is ...'
   - Use videos from Assessment Day
   - Elicit verbal feedback on progress.
10 Carers to present their child's case from first evidence of EDS difficulty to current.

11 EDS carer advice and outcome analysis. It can be useful to have a session towards the end of the day in which carers present a short talk to the group outlining their expert opinion on what essentially works and what doesn't. This helps to provide humour, develop confidence and provide peer support at a crucial time. Form 6.5 helps carers to develop their thinking in this area.

12 Course feedback: carers provide feedback to clinicians using Form 6.6.

The course co-ordinator may want to send a letter to carers prior to the Review Day to get an idea of what they would like included in the programme. This will facilitate accurate planning. At the end of each More Food Review Day, new aims for each child should be made by carers and clinicians.

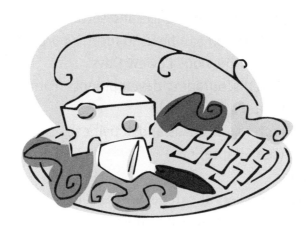

Chapter 6 Photocopiable master forms and sample forms

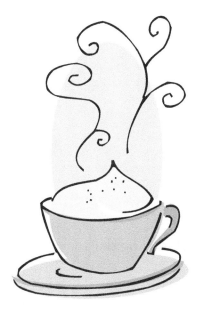

Form 6.1: Review & Performance Analysis

Name of child _____ Date _____

Carer filling in form _____ Review day No _____

1 Why did you come originally?

_____

2 Rate your original goals on a 1 to 5 scale (1 = very poor, 5 = excellent)

No.	Goal	Rating
	General progress	

3 Mark the original professional goals

No.	Goal	Rating

4 What my child did that:

Helped improve feeding skills

_____

_____

Hindered the improvement of feeding skills

_____

_____

_____

Page 1 of 2

Form 6.1: *continued*

5 What the professionals did that:

Helped improve feeding skills

_____

_____

_____

Hindered the improvement of feeding skills

_____

_____

_____

6 What carers did that:

Helped improve feeding skills

_____

_____

_____

Hindered the improvement of feeding skills

_____

_____

_____

7 What are my goals for today?

_____

_____

_____

_____

Signed _____

Form 6.2: Identifying Progress Blockers

Evaluate the time between the course/last Review Day and today and consider these questions.

1 What do you consider are the main stumbling blocks to your child's progress?

_____
_____
_____
_____
_____

2 Identify the factors which are preventing your child from making progress.

_____
_____
_____
_____
_____

3 What do you think any of us can do to help your child progress in this area?

_____
_____
_____
_____
_____

Please return your form to the course co-ordinator.

Form 6.3: Encouraging & Discouraging Developments

Name of child _____ Date _____

Carer filling in form _____ Review day No _____

Use short statements only – maximum three points

Outline any **discouraging developments** since Assessment Day:

1 _____

_____

_____

2 _____

_____

_____

3 _____

_____

_____

Outline any **encouraging developments** since Assessment Day:

1 _____

_____

_____

2 _____

_____

_____

3 _____

_____

_____

Form 6.4: Sample Statistics Feedback

Do you think your child has improved?

Here is some information from the Assessment Day to help you decide:

Eating non-preferred foods

- C ate no non-preferred foods offered
- S ate no food
- M ate no non-preferred foods
- R spent 28% of time eating non-preferred foods when offered.

Time spent sitting at table with ease

- C spent 0% of time sitting at the table with ease for non-preferred foods
- S spent 3% of time sitting at the table with ease for non-preferred foods
- M spent 0% of time sitting at the table with ease
- R spent 100% of time sitting at the table with ease.

Place of food contact

- C touched non-preferred food with her hand
- S did not make any physical contact with food
- M ate preferred food but made no bodily contact with non-preferred food
- R swallowed food offered.

Tastes & Textures

- C tasted only salty and sweet food – didn't eat any
- S & R had only experienced two tastes
- M had experienced no tastes.

Oral motor skills

Normalisation to touch – on face and inside mouth

- C tolerated no touch to her face
- R tolerated touch briefly on his cheeks only
- S & M did not tolerate touch to face or mouth.

Nutritional

- S & M were 100% tube fed
- C would drink only one liquid and eat no food
- R was slightly underweight and intake of calcium and vitamin D was poor.

Form 6.5: EDS Outcome Analysis

Your name _____ Date _____

Name of child _____

Identify three things you did that helped with EDS progress.

1 _____

2 _____

3 _____

Identify three things your child did that helped with EDS progress.

1 _____

2 _____

3 _____

Identify three things you did that hindered your child's EDS progress.

1 _____

2 _____

3 _____

Identify three things your child did that hindered his/her EDS progress.

1 _____

2 _____

3 _____

Now we want you to advise the other carers in the group. You are an expert in what not to do and what to do. Act in this capacity to advise carers new to the area. Get ready to stand up and share your skills!

Please return your form to the course co-ordinator.

Form 6.6: Review Day Feedback Form

1 Would you do the course again? ☐ Yes ☐ No

2 What was/were the best things about the course?

_____

_____

_____

3 What was/were the worst things about the course?

_____

_____

_____

4 What changes would you make?

_____

_____

_____

5 Would you recommend this course to a friend? ☐ Yes ☐ No

6 What aspects of the course required the most change from you?

_____

_____

_____

7 What aspects of the course required the most change from your child?

_____

_____

_____

Page 1 of 2

Form 6.6: *continued*

8 During the last session you revisited your aims from Day 1 of the course.

(a) Did you achieve what you set out to? ☐ Yes ☐ No

_____

_____

_____

(b) Do you think now that your expectations were realistic? ☐ Yes ☐ No

_____

_____

_____

9 Any other comments?

_____

_____

_____

_____

_____

Thank you for working with us, and good luck!

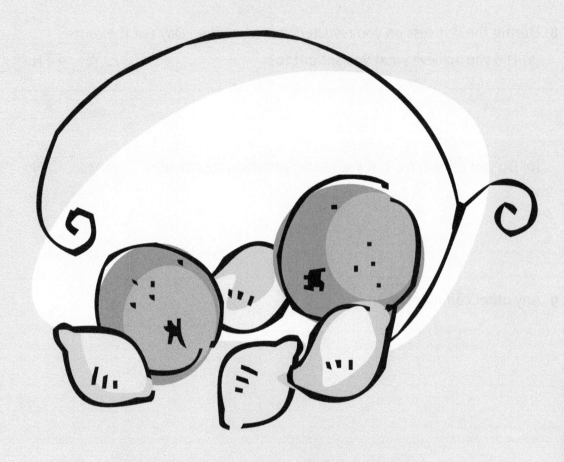

Appendices

Appendix 1: **Sample Timetables**

I Staff rota (Form A1.1)

It is always useful to organise a staff rota when utilising more than a few staff. It ensures that the day runs smoothly and that staff are fully aware of their roles – including which sessions they are to lead, and which sessions they are to support. Allocating preparation time to the staff members who are activity leaders is also useful.

The staff rota can be drafted onto a blank of the general timetable for the day. A sample is given on page 256.

II Assessment Day timetable (Form A1.2)

Depending on the number of children on the waiting list, the team may want to run between one and two Assessment Days. It is recommended that at least thirty minutes be given to each section of the assessment, given the depth of information required, numbers of staff and children involved, and the traffic required between various assessment rooms. Use of a co-ordinator is recommended to ensure timekeeping. Both families and team members should be reminded at the beginning of the day of the importance of adhering to the timetable. A sample is given on page 257.

III Food for Thought carer day timetable (Form A1.3)

The timetable on page 258 is only a sample, as some sessions are optional (eg Food memories) while others, such as Interaction, are essential and require a decent time allocation to facilitate proper discussion and education. Sessions which cannot be accommodated on this day can be fitted into either the Fun before Food programme or the EDS programme if necessary.

IV Fun before Food: The pre-feeding programme (Form A1.4)

A timetable should be somewhat flexible, and this is especially the case with the Fun before Food timetable which, given the intensive nature of the programme, may require changes if it is to respond effectively to the needs of the children.

Some sessions should run logically in sequence; most specifically, Oral Motor Skills should follow on from the Sensory Integration activity. A sample timetable can be found on page 259.

V EDS programme (Form A1.5)

A sample is given on page 260.

VI More Food Review Day timetable (Form A1.6)

Most More Food Review Day timetables follow the same pattern – a sample is given on page 261.

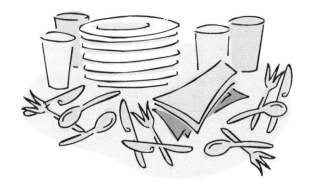

Form A1.1: Sample Staff Rota

Time	Wednesday	Thursday	Friday	Monday	Tuesday
Activity **9.30**	Orientation Lead *Name*	Weigh-in Lead *Name* Prep *Name*	Weigh-in Lead *Name* Prep *Name*	Weigh-in Lead *Name* Prep *Name*	Weigh-in Lead *Name* Prep *Name*
Activity **10.00**	EDS Lead *Name* Prep *Name*	EDS Lead *Name* Prep *Name*	EDS Lead *Name* Prep *Name*	EDS Lead *Name* Prep *Name*	EDS Lead *Name* Prep *Name*
Activity **10.45**	Carer support Lead *Name*	Carer support Lead *Name*	Carer support Lead *Name*	Carer support Lead *Name*	Carer support Lead *Name*

Form A1.2: Sample Assessment Day Timetable

Date: _____

Staff name:	AMcC	JM	GMcG	PV	CN	JOK	TM
Area	Videotaped EDS session	Sensory	Nutrition	Oral-motor	Medical	Carer support	Tastes & Textures
Room	SLT 5	OT group	Dietetics	SLT 2	Consultants 1	SLT 1	SLT 3
9.30	Stephen	George	Luke	Rory	Donal	Colin	Megan
10.00	George	Luke	Donal	Cary	Colin	Megan	Rory
10.30	Megan	Rory	Colin	Luke	Stephen	Cary	Donal
11.00	*Break*						
11.15	Cary	Stephen	George	Megan	Luke	Rory	Colin
11.45	Colin	Donal	Rory	Stephen	Megan	George	Cary
12.15	Luke	Cary	Megan	George	Rory	Donal	Stephen
12.45	*Lunch break*						
1.30	Rory	Colin	Stephen	Donal	Cary	Luke	George
2.00	Donal	Megan	Cary	Colin	George	Stephen	Luke
2.30	Carers' Q & A						
3.00	Staff meet						

Note: In the interests of accurate assessments, the videotaped individual EDS session will be an actual feeding time – plan your meal in advance and bring the relevant food and drink. Please try to ensure that, while your child is not starving, they are not too full to eat as they normally would.

Form A1.3: Sample Food for Thought Carer Day Timetable

Time	Session title	Lead
9.30	Outline of course, and rationale & carer pack	Co-ordinator
10.00	Nutrition lecture	Dietitian
10.30	Normal feeding development	SLT
11.00	Break	
11.15	Interaction	SLT
12.15	Behaviour	Psychologist/SLT
12.45	Lunch	
13.30	Therapy tips	Co-ordinator
14.00	Worst-case scenario	Psychologists
14.30	Experiential eating	SLT
15.00	Goal setting	Co-ordinator
16.00	Carer aims	Co-ordinator
16.30	Close	

Form A1.4: Fun before Food Sample Timetable

Date _____

Time	Monday	Tuesday	Wednesday
10.15	Sensory Integration	Sensory Integration	Sensory Integration
11.00	Break		
11.15	Oral Motor Skills	Oral Motor Skills	Oral Motor Skills
12.00	Growing Big & Strong	Growing Big & Strong	Growing Big & Strong
12.30	Lunch		
13.00	Normalisation	Normalisation	Normalisation
13.45	Food Play	Food Play	Food Play
14.30	Eating & Drinking & Swallowing books	Eating & Drinking & Swallowing books	Eating & Drinking & Swallowing books
15.00	Key-worker meeting	Key-worker meeting	Key-worker meeting

Form A 1.5: Sample EDS Programme Timetable

Date: _____

Time	Wednesday	Thursday	Friday	Weekend Break	Monday	Tuesday
8.15	Review progress	Review progress	Review progress		Review progress	Review progress
8.45	Goal setting	Goal setting	Goal setting		Goal setting	Goal setting
9.00	EDS BREAKFAST	EDS BREAKFAST	EDS BREAKFAST		EDS BREAKFAST	EDS BREAKFAST
9.30	Weigh-in	Weigh-in	Weigh-in		Weigh-in	Weigh-in
9.45	Identify/revisit aims	Progress evaluations	Progress evaluations		Progress evaluations	Progress evaluations
	Concurrent child session	Concurrent child session	Concurrent child session		Concurrent child session	Concurrent child session
10.15	Goal setting	Goal setting	Goal setting		Goal setting	Goal setting
10.30	EDS SNACK	EDS SNACK	EDS SNACK		EDS SNACK	EDS SNACK
11.00		*Break time*		Weekend Break		
11.15	Carer support group	Carer support group	Carer support group		Carer support group	Carer support group
	Concurrent child session	Concurrent child session	Concurrent child session		Concurrent child session	Concurrent child session
12.00	Goal setting	Goal setting	Goal setting		Goal setting	Goal setting
12.15	EDS LUNCH	EDS LUNCH	EDS LUNCH		EDS LUNCH	EDS LUNCH
12.45	Key-worker meeting	Key-worker meeting	Key-worker meeting		Key-worker meeting	Key-worker meeting
	Concurrent child session	Concurrent child session	Concurrent child session		Concurrent child session	Concurrent child session
13.15	Goal setting	Goal setting	Goal setting		Goal setting	Goal setting
13.30	EDS DESSERT	EDS DESSERT	EDS DESSERT		EDS DESSERT	EDS DESSERT
14.00	Homework planning	Homework planning	Homework planning		Homework planning	Homework planning

Form A1.6: Sample More Food Review Day Timetable

Date _____   Review Day No _____

Time	Ciara	Ronan	Luke	George	Mathilda
8.45	Goals setting				
9.00	EDS breakfast				
9.30	Feedback & group review of goals/aims				
Assessments					
10.30	Videotaped EDS session	Tastes & Textures	Nutrition	Sensory	Oral Motor Skills
11.00	Oral Motor Skills	Nutrition	Sensory	Videotaped EDS session	Tastes & Textures
11.30	Tastes & Textures	Sensory	Videotaped EDS session	Oral Motor Skills	Nutrition
12.00	Sensory	Oral Motor Skills	Tastes & Textures	Nutrition	Videotaped EDS session
12.30	Nutrition	Videotaped EDS session	Oral Motor Skills	Tastes & Textures	Sensory
13.00	EDS Lunch				
13.30	Review of Assessment Day Videos				
14.00	Carer Support Group				
14.30	EDS Dessert				
15.00	Setting Goals & Future Planning				

Note 1: Carers – please note that in the interests of accurate assessments, the videotaped individual EDS session will once again be an actual feeding time. Remember to plan your meal in advance and bring the relevant food and drink. Please try to ensure that, while your child is not starving, they are not too full to eat as they normally would.

Note 2: For the Feedback session you will be expected to give a summary of your own and your child's progress from prior to the Assessment Day to current. Your comments can be about what you think is relevant and do not need to be comprehensive. The aim is to review your own and your child's journey, and help to forward plan.

Note 3: Timekeeping is essential to ensure that everyone gets through all the elements of the programme. Please keep a close eye on the clock on the day.

Appendix 2: **Sample Reports**

I Course Report (up to the end of the EDS programme) Form A2.1)

The course report includes discussion of all elements and is largely self-explanatory. Some examples are given below.

Background section

- When the child first attended the EDS Clinic
- Who the child was referred by
- Presenting diagnosis & medical conditions
- Nutritional, medical & feeding history investigations and status
- Medications
- Previous EDS treatments
- Specific reason for placement on course.

Definition of Eating & Drinking & Swallowing problems

The definition of EDS problems should include an outline of EDS issues in all areas assessed and a summary relating to the presence of aversion, how it is typified and the level of aversion. A course report master form can be found on pages 264–68.

II End of Course Summary Note (Form A2.2)

This End of Course summary note can be used after completion of the full programme including More Food Review Days – that is, at completion of treatment. A master form can be found on pages 269–71.

III Sample reports (Forms A2.3 and A2.4)

Course report

A sample report appears on pages 272–76 and a sample summary note appears on pages 277–81.

IV Identification of aims (Forms A2.5 to A2.8)

Four sample forms appear on pages 282–85.

V Sample Sensory Profile Summary (Form A2.9)

A sample sensory profile appears on pages 286–87.

Form A2.1: Course Report Master

Re _____ **Date** _____

Address _____

DOB _____ **Chronological age** _____

The Fun with Food programme is an intensive interdisciplinary course composed of an Assessment Day, Fun before Food pre-feeding programme and an Eating & Drinking & Swallowing programme. Review Days follow the programmes. The primary focus is on developing oral eating & drinking skills in children with aversion to eating or to elements of eating & drinking. The three broad aims of the course are:

1 Education – to help carers gain a broader understanding of issues around eating & drinking skills and provide strategies to help improve skills in this area.
2 Application – to provide opportunities for carers to practise strategies under guidance and to give repeated opportunities to children to develop eating & drinking skills in peer situations.
3 Support – to give carers opportunities to share ideas, issues and concerns with others who are in a similar situation.

Team members

Clinicians _____

_____

_____

_____

Carers _____

_____

_____

Child _____

Form A2.1: *continued*

Background

Definition of Eating & Drinking & Swallowing problems/Problem identification

The range of issues affecting oral eating and drinking skills were assessed by a variety of clinicians on the Assessment Day on ＿＿＿＿＿＿＿＿＿＿＿＿＿ .

In summary:

Aims

At course commencement, the aims laid out by carers and clinicians were as identified below.

Carer ＿＿＿＿＿＿＿＿＿＿＿＿＿＿＿＿＿＿＿＿＿＿＿＿＿＿＿＿＿＿＿＿＿＿＿

Clinician ＿＿＿＿＿＿＿＿＿＿＿＿＿＿＿＿＿＿＿＿＿＿＿＿＿＿＿＿＿＿＿＿＿

Form A2.1: *continued*

Name of key-worker assigned _____

Food for Thought carer programme

This part of the programme focused on carer education and parent support and was held on the following day: _____

_____

_____

_____

_____

_____

_____

_____

Fun before Food pre-feeding programme

The Fun before Food pre-feeding programme took place on the following dates: _____. The aim of this element of the programme is to facilitate the development of skills which are important in supporting the further development of EDS skills.

Normalisation _____

_____

Oral Motor Skills _____

_____

Food Play _____

_____

Sensory Skills _____

_____

Form A2.1: *continued*

Growing Big & Strong

Eating & Drinking & Swallowing programme

The EDS programme focused on continued carer support and EDS practice, as well as on behaviour and interaction around feeding. It was held on the following dates:

Eating & Drinking & Swallowing summary

Nutritional support summary

Carer & clinician goal ratings

Carers rated aims made by both clinical staff and themselves as outlined previously.

Goals achieved: % of carer aims

                % of clinical staff aims

Goals not achieved and why

Goals achieved and why

Form A2.1: *continued*

Summary

_____

_____

_____

_____

_____

Recommendations

Name of key contact assigned _____

Action: review at More Food Review Day 1 – date: _____

Nutrition recommendations _____

_____

EDS recommendations _____

_____

Pre-feeding recommendations _____

_____

Other recommendations _____

_____

Signed by _____

Position _____

On behalf of the Fun with Food team

Cc: *EDS file*

   Department files

   Carers

   Referral source

Form A2.2: End of Course Summary Note Master

Re _____ **DOB** _____

Address _____

Fun with Food programme attendance

Programme element	Date	Attendance
Assessment Day		
Fun before Food		
Eating & Drinking & Swallowing programme		
Review Day 1		
Review Day 2		
Review Day 3		
Review Day 4		

Summary of progress

	Assessment Day	Review Day 4
Nutrition		
Interaction		
EDS		
Sensory		

Form A2.2: *continued*

Summary of progress *(continued)*

	Assessment Day	Review Day 4
Oral Motor Skills		
Tastes & Textures		

Initial aims

Initial aims from the beginning of the programme, and ratings of achievement of aims by carers, where: 1 = 0%, 2 = 25%, 3 = 50%, 4 = 75%, 5 = 100%

Clinical staff aims	Rating	Carer aims	Rating

Form A2.2: *continued*

Contact numbers

Name	Number
Dietitian	
Occupational therapist	
Speech & language therapist	
Social worker	
Psychologist	
Paediatrician	

Signed by Fun with Food course co-ordinator _____

Cc: Carer

    Referral source

    Team members

Form A2.3: Sample Course Report

Re Lucy   **Chronological age** 5 years, 7 months

Background

Lucy first attended the EDS clinic for assessment 3/12/02 when she displayed aversion to elements of oral feeding, and delayed use of oral motor functions for eating & drinking. A period of EDS interaction therapy in the early months of 2003 was not completed and Lucy was placed on the waiting list for the current programme. Lucy presented with a limited intake in terms of the range of tastes and textures taken orally, with significant aversive responses to requests to extend the range taken. In addition, Lucy resists independent self-feeding despite no obvious physical limitations that would prevent her from using this skill.

Lucy's feeding and medical history of note include a diagnosis of Down syndrome, naso-gastric (NG) tube feeding at birth for three weeks, cardiac surgery at three months with NG tube feeding for three and a half weeks after this, a history of recurrent upper respiratory tract infections, myringotomy, and one episode of pneumonia for which she was hospitalised pre-cardiac surgery.

Problem identification

The range of issues affecting oral eating skills were assessed by a variety of clinicians on the Assessment Day on _____. In summary, Lucy presents with selective oral eating characterised by an extremely limited range of tastes and textures taken, and concomitant behavioural issues including throwing food and chairs, screaming and hitting out, crawling under the table, and running from the room. She also presents with mild oral motor dysfunction characterised by an open mouth posture and limited chewing ability. There is mild hyposensitivity and hypotonicity.

Aims

Carer

1 Highlight areas of weakness that preclude her from progressing towards normal eating

2 Learn small steps for guidance towards achieving goal

Page 1 of 5

Form A2.3: *continued*

3 Make mealtimes less of a stressful, major issue

4 Make some progress towards her chewing and eating normal food.

Clinicians

1 Manage behaviour around feeding via interaction guidelines and principles

2 Develop active participation during feeding, ie self-feeding

3 Develop textural range to include foods which require biting and chewing.

Key-worker assigned: Brian

Fun before Food pre-feeding programme

The Fun before Food programme took place two weeks before the EDS programme. The aim of this part of the programme is to facilitate the development of skills, which are important in supporting EDS skills. The programme ran over three days with an average of three sessions per activity area. Activities areas included Normalisation Strategies, Oral Motor Skills, Food Play, Sensory Skills, and Growing Big & Strong (Nutrition).

Lucy displays aversion to elements of oral feeding, and although strong behavioural elements are noted, there is also the suggestion of oral motor dysfunction. Also the Sensory Profile completed on the Assessment Day indicates some difficulties with oral sensory processing, behavioural outcomes of sensory processing, and more significant difficulty with visual processing. Lucy had made progress on Day 3 of the pre-feeding programme but was noted to have difficulties with wet textures in Food Play on Day 3. She responded well to deep pressure in the Oral Motor activities. Co-operation on tasks like making sandwiches was excellent. Generally Lucy's co-operation for non-play activities was reduced, impacting on the effectiveness of input, and she required structure and carry-over work prior to the EDS section of the programme commencing.

Eating & Drinking & Swallowing programme

The EDS part of the programme focused on parent education, parent support and eating & drinking immersion. There were a total of 18 EDS sessions, five nutritional support sessions, and four parent support sessions.

Page 2 of 5

Form A2.3: *continued*

Eating & Drinking & Swallowing:

Goals centred on compliance, with small staged goals centred on food approach behaviour (eg sitting at the table), and increasing the number of spoons taken orally by range of textures. Non-compliance behaviour reduced significantly from lengthy EDS sessions composed of Lucy repeatedly throwing utensils with food off the table and getting up from the table, to Lucy staying and accepting – within minutes – new tastes and textures, which included mixed textures. Self-feeding developed, with significantly reduced requests from Lucy to spoon-feed her. Lucy is expected to make continuing progress in EDS skills given the support of her parents and nanny who all attended with her. Suggestions made, and carried out, to reduce the amount of language directed to Lucy during feeding, restating goals and setting boundaries facilitated Lucy's progress.

Nutritional support:

Day 1

Weight: Actual Body Weight (ABW): 18kg

                 Ideal Body Weight (IBW): 18kg

                 Height (Ht): 100cm

Dietary problems: Food is finely mashed, Lucy has snacks between meals and while these are nutritious, they would not allow appetite to develop.

Day 1 evening goal: Change consistency to improve nutritional intake. Reduce number of snacks, change to calcium-enriched soya milk with added vitamin D.

Day 5

Weight: ABW 17.8kg

                 IBW 18.0kg

                 Ht 100cm

Lucy maintained weight while developing the range of foods taken orally.

Parent support:

Lucy is an only child. She has Down syndrome. Both parents work full-time and Lucy has a full-time childminder. She goes to playschool. At initial assessment, Lucy was described as eating only puréed food, was not chewing and would not tolerate finger

Form A2.3: *continued*

foods. She was said to have a broad range of tastes. When asked why they thought feeding was difficult for Lucy, her parents explained that she had some sensory issues and that she had phobias in some areas. Overall they felt that there was a psychological aspect to the problem. Feeding could be difficult every day if they persisted with introducing lumps. Also, Lucy was particular about using her own equipment, mugs, bowls and so on.

Food shopping and cooking is shared between both parents and the childminder. The childminder is currently Lucy's main feeder. Lucy will eat normally in relation to time if she is happy about the consistency of the food.

When asked about other difficulties they have concerns about, Lucy's parents spoke about Lucy's sleep pattern. She wakes at 6 am, which is an improvement on her previous time of between 4 and 5 am.

Both parents attended the programme and contributed well to the parent sessions and they discussed many areas of concern.

Parent & professional goal ratings

Lucy's parents rated aims made by both clinical staff and themselves, as outlined above. Lucy's parents felt they had achieved 95 per cent of their own aims for the course, and 80 per cent of clinical staff aims.

All goals were achieved to a degree. Lucy's food approach behaviour has improved significantly, as has her ability to accept new textures. Self-feeding by spoon is developing and finger feeding is commencing. Oral motor function to support chewing needs to be explored.

Summary

Lucy and her parents made significant strides with regard to her eating & drinking skills following a huge commitment on all their parts. Lucy is expected to continue to develop her skills in this area.

Page 4 of 5

Form A2.3: *continued*

Recommendations

1 Key contact assigned – Brian
2 Review at Review Day – end March
3 Further evaluate oral motor support for chewing
4 Encourage intake of protein foods, vary intake of vegetables
5 Take 1 _____ daily to ensure a good intake of calcium and protein.

Signed _____

Course co-ordinator

Fun with Food programme

Cc: Referral source

   Carers

   Team members

Form A2.4: End of Course Summary Note Sample

Re Marty   **Age** 8 years

Fun with Food programme attendance

Programme element	Date	Attendance
Assessment Day		✓
Fun before Food		✓
Eating & Drinking & Swallowing programme		✓
Review Day 1		✓
Review Day 2		cancelled
Review Day 3		✓

Summary of progress

	Assessment Day	Review Day 3
Nutrition	Actual body wt: 25.5kg Ideal body wt: 26kg Ht: 127.1 cm 1 Marty had a very limited intake of foods, ie six items 2 Finds it difficult to try new drinks or foods 3 Takes only sodas and calcium supplement.	Actual body wt: 26.2kg Ideal body wt: 27kg Ht: 129.6 cm 1 Marty has grown and gained weight over the past six months. He is still slightly underweight 2 His only source of protein is hard cheese and sausages 3 Now takes 25ml milk daily, but continues to drink orange, cola or lemon

Form A2.4: *continued*

Summary of progress *(continued)*

	Assessment Day	Review Day 3
Interaction Table behaviour	Preferred foods 100% sitting with ease Non-preferred foods 0% sitting with ease	Preferred foods 96% sitting with ease Non-preferred foods 96% sitting with ease
Eating behaviour	Preferred foods spent 100% of time actually eating Non-preferred foods spent 0% of time actually eating	Preferred foods spent 61% time actually eating Non-preferred foods spent 94% of time actually eating
Oral nutritional behaviour	Preferred food – 20 swallows Non-preferred foods: no touch, oral placement or swallow	Preferred food – 6 swallows Non-preferred foods: 11 swallows
Food range	Tastes: Sweet only Consistencies: liquid and mixed texture taken	Tastes: savoury and sweet tastes taken Consistencies: liquids, purées, separate lumps and mixed textures taken
EDS	EDS Day 1 Session 1 goals: 1 Will take one bite and swallow of a new biscuit – achieved 2 Will sit at table for two minutes – achieved	Review Day 3 Session 2 goals: 1 Will eat six spoons of custard – achieved 2 Will eat five chips – achieved 3 Will eat a slice of ham – achieved

Form A2.4: *continued*

Summary of progress *(continued)*

	Assessment Day	Review Day 3
Sensory	1 Marty presented with a mixed sensory profile, with his physical disability, perceptual difficulties and behaviour impacting on his performance level in activities 2 While Marty presented with some reluctance to accept tactile information around his face and mouth, main difficulties are not felt to be solely due to sensory processing problems 3 Marty also presented with significant difficulty attending to task	1 Sensory diet was recommended for home, incorporating movement, deep pressure and resistive activities 2 Mother is continuing with the sensory programme at home and finds it to be very beneficial for Marty, especially in relation to his ability to attend to task
Oral motor sensory	Tolerated touch on face only Aware of different parts of face, difficulty with discrimination inside mouth	Tolerates touch on face and in mouth with toothette and vibrator Able to tolerate three different textures in mouth simultaneously Aware of different parts of face and mouth Able to discriminate touch inside mouth

Page 3 of 5

Form A2.4: *continued*

Summary of progress *(continued)*

	Assessment Day	Review Day 3
Oral imitation	Efficient jaw grading Adequate movement and strength in lips Associated jaw movements observed during tongue movement	Efficient jaw grading Adequate movement and strength in lips Associated jaw movements observed during tongue movement
Oral motor activities	*Horn/whistle:* Poor lip closure, good tongue retraction, jaw stability and breath support *Bubbles:* Poor lip rounding and jaw stability Difficulty with airflow grading *Straw:* Lip rounding reduced tongue but retraction efficient Good co-ordination of suck–swallow–breathe *Spatula:* Inefficient lip closure and strength Jaw stability adequate for this task	Good lip closure, tongue retraction, jaw stability and breath support Efficient lip rounding and tongue retraction Difficulty with grading of airflow Lip rounding and tongue retraction efficient Good co-ordination of suck–swallow–breathe Efficient lip closure and strength Jaw stability adequate for this task
Tastes & Textures	8 foods	17 foods

Page 4 of 5

Form A2.4: *continued*

Identification of goals from end of Review Day 3

Clinical staff

1 Continue to take supplements: 1 multivitamin drop daily and calcium tablets daily

2 Continue to make small changes in tastes and textures

3 Develop food play with mashed textures

4 Marty benefits from distraction during eating, particularly, for example, pretend play toys such as trains with toy people

5 Don't use questions when feeding – gives the opportunity for refusal

6 Continue with sensory programme

7 Reschedule psychology appointment

8 Dietitian to monitor when Marty attends paediatrician

9 Review on request.

Parent

1 Food preparation and cooking sessions at least twice a week

2 Small steps when introducing new food

3 Try to improve amounts of food taken.

Signed by Fun with Food course co-ordinator _____

Cc: Carer

    Referral source

    Team members

Identification of aims, Sample 1

Form A2.5: Identification of Initial Programme Aims Food for Thought Carer Day

Name of child Cian

Clinical staff	Carer
1 Develop a structure around eating & drinking 2 Develop management of behaviour via interaction guidelines and principles 3 Increase range of textures being taken orally.	1 For Cian not to be afraid of food. To be able to taste things without having a panic attack 2 To get him to sit at a table 3 To be able to bring him to a restaurant 4 For him to be able to drink milk. He only drinks juice and it rots his teeth 5 I would really love him to eat even two extra things. This would make this course a huge success for me.

Cc: Carer

   File

Identification of aims, Sample 2

Form A2.6: Identification of Aims from End of Review Day 1 to Review Day 2

Name of child Davy

Clinical staff	Carer
1 Increase intake of wet textures	1 Eat by himself
2 Commence intake of defined lumps	2 Take more varied textures involving chewing or swallowing
3 Continue as before – increase volume of all food	
4 Increase participation in independent feeding.	

Cc: Carer

   File

Identification of aims, Sample 3

Form A2.7: Identification of Aims from End of Review Day 2 to Review Day 3

Name of child Liam

Clinical staff	Carer
1 Trial different types of stimulation for tooth grinding, eg citrus, thermal, oral motor activities, distraction etc	1 Decrease thickness of liquid – progress towards un-thickened
2 Re food cramming – identify/analyse food that encourages this, eg doughy bread etc	2 Develop cup drinking
	3 Reduce cramming behaviour
3 Re cramming, try different textures to see if this helps, eg crackers, soda bread etc	4 Stop teeth grinding by replacing stimulation
4 Trial 'Wake-Up' activities prior to eating, eg thermal stimulation as discussed	5 Continue working on independence – putting food into mouth and feeding self.
5 Let him take responsibility for cleaning self during feeding	
6 Take a second yoghurt daily	
7 Check re availability of valved cups	
8 Evaluation of spoon feeding next visit	
9 Refer to paediatrician – concern re reflux.	

Cc: Carer

   File

Identification of aims, Sample 4

Form A2.8: Review Day 4

Name of child Katy

Clinical staff	Carer
1 Manage behaviour/structure around feeding via interaction principles	1 To continue progress we have made over the last year. We are thrilled with Katy's achievement to date
2 Focus on and develop the positive aspects of feeding	2 To remove stress for Katy and to make mealtimes fun for her (and us), and something for her to look forward to
3 Develop use of drinking utensil for liquids	3 I would like Katy to be aware of hunger/smell – also to get her to try new foods
4 Evaluate nutritional intake.	4 To be independently feeding – both food and drink. I am afraid that if we did not feed Katy she would not eat/drink. We don't know how we can push this
	5 For Katy to sit with family and stay seated at mealtimes – this can sometimes be stressful and hard to enforce because of outside factors.

Comments:

The Fun with Food programme has made us more aware of the issues for Katy and why she reacts in certain ways. We hope to use the information to make more improvements.

Cc: Carer

File

Form A2.9: Sample Sensory Profile Results

You completed the Sensory Profile Questionnaire on your child at the time of the Assessment Day. Results suggest 'typical performance' in 9 out of 14 sections. However, for sections of vestibular processing and touch processing, although results indicate normal processing, observations of participation in these tasks would suggest sensory defensiveness and low threshold.

1 Your child achieved scores suggesting *'probable difference'*, that is, with potential to interfere with daily activities, in sections of:

   (a) Auditory processing
   Your child's reaction in a group/noisy situation would suggest that difficulty with processing auditory information is more significant than identified here.

   (b) Oral sensory processing
   The pattern of scores in this area suggests very low threshold for oral sensory stimuli.

   (c) Modulation of movement
   Affecting activity level due to preference for sedentary activities.

2 Your child achieved scores suggesting *'definite difference'*, that is, sensory processing difficulty likely to be interfering with daily function in sections of:

   (a) Sensory processing related to endurance/tone
   This is felt to be primarily due to physical factors.

   (b) Behavioural outcomes of sensory processing – due to:
   difficulty with colouring/writing activities.

   (c) Poor tolerance of changes in plans/routines
   There is some physical involvement here also.

Form A2.9: *continued*

While the sensory profile gives us some useful information on your child's behaviour in relation to a range of activities, it is felt that the information from individual activity and group sessions gives us a better picture of your child's sensory processing abilities.

Please do not hesitate to contact the occupational therapist _____
if you require any more information on any of the above, at _____ .

Signed _____
Fun with Food course co-ordinator
Cc: Carers
   File

Appendix 3: **Sample Letters**

Sample letters (Forms A3.1 to A3.5) that can be used in the programme follow on pages 289–94.

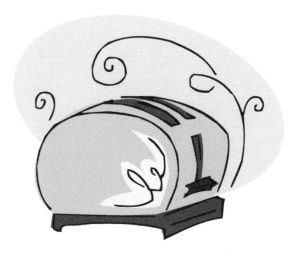

Form A3.1: Assessment Day Invitation

Date _____

Dear Carer

As some of you will know, we are holding an intensive Eating, Drinking & Swallowing course for children who are aversive to oral feeding, or to elements of oral feeding. It has three main parts:

1 **Food for Thought carers' day** for carers only
2 **Fun before Food**, which focuses on pre-feeding issues such as sensory skills, oral motor development etc, and two weeks later a five-day programme:
3 **Eating & Drinking & Swallowing**, which focuses on Eating & Drinking skills.

The course is interdisciplinary with team members from the following disciplines: speech & language therapy, dietetics, occupational therapy, social work, paediatrics and psychology.

The course dates which require the attendance of at least one carer and child on each day are as follows:

Course component	Date	Times
Assessment Day		9.30am–3.00pm
Fun before Food		8.30am–2.30pm daily
Eating & Drinking & Swallowing	(excluding weekend)	8.30am–2pm daily
Review Day 1		8.45am–3.30pm
Review Day 2		8.45am–3.30pm
Review Day 3		8.45am–3.30pm
Review Day 4		8.45am–3.30pm

Your child has been selected as a *possible* candidate. In order to demonstrate your interest, to confirm you will attend the Assessment Day, and are available if chosen for the course to attend *all* the dates noted above, please fill in the confirmation form below and return by _____ to the course co-ordinator.

Signed _____

Course coordinator

Page 1 of 2

Form A3.1: *continued*

CONFIRMATION FORM

☐ Would you be interested in coming?

☐ Could both carers come?

☐ Can you attend the Assessment Day?

☐ Can you attend the Fun before Food and Fun with Food intensive courses?

☐ Can you attend the Review days?

Name of child

Address

Carer's signature

Contact number/s

Form A3.2: Assessment Day Timetable

Date _____

Dear Carer

Please find enclosed the Assessment Day timetable for you and your child. As times are tight, please try to keep to the timetable to ensure complete assessments for all children.

We will have a Carer Meeting in the early afternoon to outline the course itself and answer any initial questions you may have.

Please note that at the end of the day the team will meet to discuss the children who attended for assessment. A maximum of _____ children will be offered a place on the course based on their individual needs, and how the group will fit together. Those children who are not offered a place will be kept on the list and reconsidered for the next course.

We will contact you a few days after your child's assessment with the team to let you know.

We have enclosed questionnaires and forms for you to fill in. We realise this is a lot of work for you but it will help to ensure a thorough assessment for your child and make the process more efficient. Please bring your forms with you on the day and give them to the course co-ordinator, who is _____.

On the day of assessment please bring at least one solid and one drink that your child will accept relatively easily, and one solid and one drink they refuse – perhaps foods you have tried with your child without success. If there are no foods your child will take, do not worry. Please bring some foods anyway.

If you have any queries please phone _____.

Looking forward to seeing you on the day.

Signed _____
Course co-ordinator

Form A3.3: Offer Letter

Date _____

Dear Carer

Your child _____ has been offered a place as discussed on the phone with you.

The dates are as follows.
Fun before Food:
From _____ to _____ Time 8.30–2.30pm
Eating & Drinking & Swallowing:
From _____ to _____ Time 8.30–2.00pm
The Food for Thought carer day will be held on _____, starts at 9.00am, and is held in _____.
This is a day for carers only – do not bring your child.

Please find enclosed preliminary timetables for the programme sections Fun before Food and Eating & Drinking & Swallowing.

We would be grateful if you would confirm your attendance within the next week. If you are unable to attend please let us know as soon as possible so we can offer your child's place to another child.

It will be an intensive programme, but there is a break for lunch, at least!
Your child has a key-worker allocated to them who is: _____.

Please bring a change of clothes, as some of the activities can be quite messy. Wipes and cloths may also be useful. We look forward to seeing you on the

_____.

Please contact _____ if you have any queries.
Looking forward to working with you

Signed _____
Course co-ordinator

Form A3.4: Review Day No: ＿＿ Letter

Date ＿＿＿＿＿＿＿＿＿＿＿＿＿

Dear Carers

As you know Review Day No ＿＿＿ is to take place on ＿＿＿＿＿＿＿＿＿＿＿＿＿ .
We will attempt to organise a timetable that fits both with your needs and our aims,
and will forward the timetable to you nearer the time. To facilitate planning, please fill
in the enclosed slip and return it by surface post or email by ＿＿＿＿＿＿＿＿＿＿＿ .
I appreciate your help in this and look forward to seeing you soon.
Take care.

Signed ＿＿＿＿＿＿＿＿＿＿＿＿＿
Course co-ordinator

Fun with Food Review Day number ▮▮▮

Name of child ＿＿＿＿＿＿＿＿＿＿＿＿ Date ＿＿＿＿＿＿＿＿＿＿＿＿

I would like you to include these activities in the joint review day:

1 ＿＿＿

2 ＿＿＿

3 ＿＿＿

These are my goals for my child on the joint review day:

1 ＿＿＿

2 ＿＿＿

3 ＿＿＿

Additional comments:

＿＿＿

＿＿＿

＿＿＿

＿＿＿

Form A3.5: End of Course Letter

Date _____

Dear Carer

The programme is finally finished! We hope you have both enjoyed and learned from your experience with us, and that we have added to your skills to enable you to take your child's eating and drinking skills forward.

I have just finished looking through the re-assessment videos and it was a pleasant experience! In addition to the improvements made by all the children over the course of the programme, what was most noticeable was the carers' and children's relaxed manner and relative ease around the process of eating and drinking. This was a huge step for everyone, so well done. Also, praise and reinforcement of your children's achievements was highly evident and the children responded well to these strategies.

On behalf of the team I would like to thank you all for all the effort and very hard work that you have put in. This, and your open and constant support of each other, was the cornerstone of your child's progress. You and your children have all done brilliantly, and we hope you are happy with your progress.

Enclosed is a summary report and our agreed goals from the last day of the course. Included in the report are contact numbers for the members of staff if you need any further help or advice or just get stuck. Please keep us informed of how you are getting on.

Remember to always have clear goals. This will continue to help you and your child to move forward.

Good luck!

Signed _____
Course co-ordinator

Appendix 4: **Carer Comments**

- The Fun before Food programme has made us more aware of the issues for George, and why he reacts in certain ways. We hope to use the information to make more improvements. It is lovely to get golden moments, eg George, head stuck in fridge, or this week – George touching his face parts with food and naming them.

- A most intense but worthwhile week.

- Expectations were surpassed.

- Thank you so much. You made such a difference to Carl's life and our family life.

- An invaluable course that any carer who has a child with feeding problems should have access to.

- Great learning process.

- Found the course gave us great confidence to set boundaries with regard to feeding and other aspects of life.

Weigh-in

- Good to know not losing weight while trying new foods.

Goal setting

- Found the course gave us great confidence to set new boundaries with regard to feeding and also other aspects of life.

- Breaking issues into capable portions.

- Very helpful, principles definitely worked for my child.

- Allowed carers to be in control and set their own goals.

Carer needs

- Was great to talk to carers with the same problem.

- We were all in the same boat.

- Met individual needs and allowed for questions.

- The removal of the children when discussing/thinking was required was great.

- Great respect and acknowledgement of carers.

- Overall a real model of parent–professional partnership.

- As carers we learned a lot.

- Freedom to talk and listen.

The best things about the programme

- Meeting other people with the same problems.

- My child was looked at from a number of issues affecting feeding – a good global approach.

- Videos – seeing how we progressed.

- Professional support and advice.

- Team approach.

- Support among carers.

Aspects requiring most change for carers

- Keeping emotion out of food.

- Learning to set goals – which removes stress and panic.

- Having higher expectations for my child.

- Gaining confidence to push Lucy into eating.

Aspects requiring most change for children according to carers

- Trying new foods.

- Learning to trust clinician's word.

- Knowing we expected goals to be met.

- Acceptance of rules.

- Eating lumpier foods.

Bibliography

Abrahams P & Burkitt BFE, 1970, 'Hiatus hernia and gastro-oesophageal reflux in children with cerebral palsy', *Australian Pediatric Journal*, 6, p41.

Alexander R, 1987, 'Prespeech & Feeding Development', McDonald ET (ed), *Treating Cerebral Palsy: For Clinicians by Clinicians*, pp133–52, Pro-ed, Austin, TX.

Ayres AJ, 1979, '*Sensory Integration and the Child*', Western Psychological Services, Los Angeles, CA.

Babbit RL, Hoch TA & Coe DA, 1994. 'Behavioural Feeding Disorders', Tuchman DN & Walter RS (eds), *Disorders of Feeding and Swallowing in Infants and Children*, pp77–96, Singular Publishing, San Diego, CA.

Bax MCO, 1989, 'Eating is important', *Developmental Medicine and Child Neurology* 31, pp285–6.

Bayer LM, Bauers CM & Kapp SR, 1983, 'Psychosocial aspects of nutritional support', *Nursing Clinics of North America* 1, pp119–28.

Benda GIM, 1979, 'Modes of Feeding Low-Birth-Weight Infants', *Seminars in Perinatology* 3 (4), pp407–15.

Benoit D, Wang EE & Slotkin SH, 2000, 'Discontinuation of enterostomy tube feeding by behavioural intervention for a child with chronic food refusal and gastrostomy tube dependence', *Journal of Pediatrics* 137 (4), pp498–503.

Blackman JA, 1998, 'Children who refuse food', *Contemporary Pediatrics* 15 (10), pp198–216.

Boyle JT, 1991, 'Nutritional management of the developmentally disabled child', *Pediatric Surgery International* 6, pp76–81.

Boshart C, 1998, *Oral-Motor Analysis and Remediation Techniques,* Speech Dynamics Inc, Temecula, CA.

Brazelton TB, 1979, 'Neonatal Behavioural Assessment Scale', *Clinics in Developmental Medicine* No. 50, Lippincott, Philadelphia, PA.

Bundy A, 1991, 'Assessing Sensory Integrative Dysfunction', Bundy A, Lane S & Murray E (eds), S*ensory Integration: Theory and Practice*, 2nd edn, FA Davis Company, Philadelphia, PA.

Bundy A & Murray E, 1991, 'Sensory Integration: Jean Ayres' Theory Revisited', Bundy A, Lane S & Murray E (eds), *Sensory Integration: Theory and Practice,* 2nd edn, FA Davis Company, Philadelphia, PA.

Bundy A, Lane S & Murray E, 1991, S*ensory Integration: Theory and Practice*, 2nd edn, FA Davis Company, Philadelphia, PA.

Byars KC, Burklow KA, Ferguson K, O'Flaherty T, Santoro K & Kaula A, 2003, 'A Multicomponent Behavioural program for oral aversion in children dependent on gastrostomy feedings', *Journal of Pediatric Gastrostomy and Nutrition* 37, pp473–80.

Byrne WJ, Euler AR, Ashcraft E, Nash DG, Seibert JJ & Golladay ES, 1982, 'Gastro-oesophageal reflux in the severely retarded who vomit: Criteria for and results of surgical intervention in twenty two patients', *Surgery* 91, pp95–98.

Carroll L & Reilly S, 1996, 'The therapeutic approach to the child with feeding difficulty: Management and Treatment', Sullivan P & Rosenbloom L (eds), *Feeding The Disabled Child*, MacKeith Press, London, pp117–31.

Case-Smith J, Cooper P & Scala V, 1989, 'Feeding Behaviour in pre-term neonates', *American Journal of Occupational Therapy* 43 (4), pp245–50.

Case-Smith J, 2001, *Occupational Therapy for Children*, 4th edn, Mosby, St Louis, MO.

Casear D, Daniels H, Develieger H, De Cock P & Eggermont E, 1982, 'Feeding Behaviour in pre-term neonates', *Early Human Development* 7, pp331–46.

Cataldi-Betcher EL, Seltzer MH, Slocum BA & Jones KW, 1983, 'Complications occurring during enteral nutrition support: a prospective study', *Journal of Parenteral and Enteral Nutrition* 7 (6), pp546–52.

Chapman Bahr D, 2001, *Oral motor assessment and treatment: Ages and Stages,* Allen & Bacon, Needham Heights, MA.

Christophen ER & Hall CC, 1978, 'Eating Pattern and Associated Problems encountered in Normal Children', *Issues in Comprehensive Paediatric Nursing* 17, pp81–94.

Cocks A, 2000, *Nutritional requirements for Children in Health and Disease*, 3rd edn, Great Ormond Street Hospital for Children NHS Trust, London.

Colodny N, 2001, 'Construction and validation of the mealtime and dysphagia questionnaire: an instrument designed to assess nursing staff reasons for noncompliance with SLP dysphagia and feeding recommendations', *Dysphagia*, 16 (4), pp263–71.

Cooke RW, 1994, 'Factors effecting survival and outcome at three years in extremely preterm infants', *Archives of Diseases in Childhood* 71, pp28–31.

Copeland M & Kimmel J, 1989, *Evaluation and Management of Infants and Young Children with Developmental Disabilities,* Brookes publishing, Baltimore, MD.

Dello Strologo L, Principato F, Sinibaldi D, Appiani AC, Terzi F, Dartois AM & Rizzoni G, 1997, 'Feeding dysfunction in infants with severe chronic renal failure after long-term naso-gastric tube feeding', *Pediatric Nephrology* 11, pp84–86.

Dobie RA, 1978, 'Rehabilitation of swallowing disorders', *American Family Physician* 27, pp84–95.

Doyle Morrison C & Metzger P, 2001, Case-Smith J (ed), *Occupational Therapy for Children*, 4th edn, Mosby, St Louis, MO.

Dunn W, 1997, 'The Impact of Sensory Processing Abilities on the Daily Lives of Young Children and Their Families: A Conceptual Model', *Infants and Young Children* 9 (4), pp23–35.

Dunn W, 1999a, *Sensory Profile: Caregiver questionnaire,* Psychological Corporation, San Antonio, TX.

Dunn W, 1999b, *Sensory Profile: Users Manual,* Psychological Corporation, San Antonio, TX.

Dunn Klein M & Evans Morris S, 1999, *Mealtime Participation Guide,* Therapy Skill Builders, San Antonio, TX.

Epping Forest Primary Care Trust, Nutrition & Dietetics Department, *Teddy: Fun Food Pack,* Epping Essex.

Erenberg A & Nowak AJ, 1984, 'Appliances for stabilising orogastric and orotracheal tubes in infants', *Critical Care Medicine* 12, pp669–71.

Evans Morris S & Dunn Klein M, 1987, *Prefeeding Skills,* Therapy Skill Builders, Tucson, AZ.

Farrell DA, Hagopian LP & Kurtz PF, 2001, 'A hospital and home-based behavioural intervention for a child with chronic food refusal and gastrostomy tube dependence', *Journal of Developmental and Physical Disabilities* 13 (4), pp407–18.

Ferry GD, Selby M, & Pietro TJ, 1983, 'Clinical response to short term naso-gastric feeding in infants with gastro-oesophageal reflux and growth failure', *Journal of Paediatric Gastroenterology and Nutrition* 2, pp57–61.

Frick SM, Frick R, Oetter P & Richter E, 1996, *'Out of the Mouths of Babes: Discovering the Developmental Significance of the Mouth',* PDP Press Inc, Stillwater, MN.

Gadenstatter M, Wykypiel H, Schwab GP, Profanter C, & Wetscher GJ, 1999, 'Respiratory symptoms and dysphagia in patients with gastro-oesophageal reflux disease: a comparison of medical and surgical therapy', *Langenbeck's Archives of Surgery* 384(6), pp563–7.

Gessell A, 1940, *The first five years of life: A guide to the study of the preschool child*, Harper & Brothers, New York, NY.

Gisel E, 1994, 'Oral-motor skills following sensorimotor intervention in the moderately eating-impaired child with CP', *Dysphagia* 9 (3), pp180–92.

Gisel EG & Patrick J, 1998, 'Identification of children with cerebral palsy unable to maintain a normal nutritional state', *Lancet* 1, pp283–6.

Gisel EG, Applegate-Ferrante T, Benson JE & Bosma JF, 1995, 'Effects of oral sensorimotor treatment on measures of growth and eating efficiency and aspiration in the dysphagic child with CP', *Developmental Medicine and Child Neurology* 37 (6), pp528–43.

Gisel EG, Applegate-Ferrante T, Benson J & Bosma JF, 1996, 'Oral motor skills following sensorimotor therapy in two groups of moderately dysphagic children with CP: aspiration vs. non aspiration', *Dysphagia* 11 (1), pp59–71.

Gisel EK, Tessier MJ, Lapierre G, Seidman E, Drouin E & Filion G, 2003, 'Feeding management of children with severe CP and eating impairment: an exploratory study', *Physical & Occupational Therapy in Pediatrics* 23 (2), pp19–44.

Guttentag S & Hammer D, 2000, 'Shaping oral feeding in a gastrostomy tube-dependent child in natural settings', *Behavior Modification* 24 (3), pp395–410.

Hancock J, 1995, 'The effects of prematurity on long term outcome', *Paediatric Nursing* 7 (10), pp14–19.

Handen BL, Mandell F & Russo DC, 1986, 'Feeding induction in children who refuse to eat', *American Journal of Diseases in Childhood* 140, pp52–54.

Harris G, 2000, Paper presented at the Focus on Feeding Conference, Dublin.

Helfrish-Miller KR, Rector KL & Straka JA, 1986, 'Dysphagia: its treatment in the profoundly retarded patient with cerebral palsy', *Archives of Physical and Medical Rehabilitation* 67 (8), pp520–5.

Huggins PS, Tuomi SK & Young C, 1999, 'Effects of Naso-gastric Tubes on the Young Normal Swallowing Mechanism', *Dysphagia* 14, pp157–61.

Jared J, Boshart C, Demetrion H, Kelly L, Haislip C, Schueller M, Harrison T & Szypulski T, 2000, *Great therapy ideas! Oral Sensory-Motor Tool-Toys Techniques,* Speech Dynamics Inc, Temecula, CA.

Jones TW, 1982, 'Treatment of behaviour related eating problems in retarded students: A review of the literature', Hollis JH & Meyers CE (eds), *Life threatening behaviour: Analysis and Intervention,* American Association of Mental Deficiency, Washington, DC.

Kerwin ML, Jefferson G & Geecher J, May 1992, *Evaluation of the effectiveness of oral stimulation for promoting oral-motor skills and food acceptance,* Paper presented at meeting of association for behaviour analysts, San Francisco, CA (web address: www.jeibi.com).

Kinnealy, M, Oliver B & Wilbarger P, 1995, 'A Phenomenological Study of Sensory Defensiveness in Adults', *American Journal of Occupational Therapy* 49 (5), pp444–51.

Klein MD & Delaney T, 1994, *Feeding and Nutrition for the Child with Special Needs,* Therapy Skills Builders, Tucson, AZ.

Koontz Lowman D & McKeever Murphy S, 1999, *The Educator's Guide to Feeding Children with Disabilities,* Paul H Brookes Publishing Co, Philiadelphia, PA.

Krick J & VanDuyn MAS, 1984, 'The relationship between oral motor involvement and growth – A pilot study in a pediatric population with cerebral palsy', *Journal of the American Dietetic Association* 84 (5), pp555–69.

Krick J, Murphy PE, Markham J & Shapiro BK, 1991, 'A Proposed Formula for calculating energy needs of children with Cerebral Palsy', *Developmental Medicine & Child Neurology* 43: pp481–7.

Krick J, Murphy-Miller PE, Zeger S & Wright E, 1996, 'Patterns of Growth in Children with Cerebral Palsy', *Journal of the American Dietetic Association* 96 (7),pp680–5.

Linscheid TR, 1978, 'Disturbance of eating and feeding', Magreb PM (ed), *Psychological management of Pediatric problems: Early Life conditions and chronic diseases Vol 1,* University Park Press, Baltimore, MD.

Luiselli JK, 1989, 'Behavioural assessment and treatment of pediatric feeding disorders in developmental disabilities', Hersen M, Eisler RM, & Miller PM (eds), *Progress in Behaviour Modification Vol 24,* pp91–131, Sage, Newbury Park, CA.

Macky E, 1996, *Oral Motor Activities for Young Children,* LinguiSystems Inc, IL.

Marshalla P, 2001, *Oral Motor Techniques in Articulation & Phonological Therapy,* Marshalla Speech and Language, Kirkland, WA.

Mathews S, Williams R & Pring T, 1997, 'Parent–child interaction therapy and dysfluency: a single case study', *European Journal of Disorders of Communication* 32, pp346–57.

Mathisen B, Skuse D, Wolke D & Reilly S, 1999, 'Oral motor dysfunction and failure to thrive among inner city infants', *Developmental Medicine and Child Neurology* 31, pp293–302.

McCance & Widdowson S, 2002, *The Composition of Foods,* Sixth Summary Edn, Royal Society of Chemistry, Cambridge.

McCurtin A, 1997, *The Manual of Paediatric Feeding Practice,* Speechmark Publishing, Bicester.

McCurtin A, Kennedy M & Kelly G, 'Factors predictive of, or associated with aversive oral feeding'. (Unpublished)

McCurtin A, Kennedy M & Walsh C, 'Interdisciplinary treatment programme for selective and total aversive oral feeders'. (Unpublished)

McInnes JM & Treffney JA, 1982, *Deaf–Blind Infants and Children: A Developmental Guide,* University of Toronto Press, Toronto.

McKeever Murphy S & Caretto V, 1997, 'Anatomy of the Oral and Respiratory Structures made Easy', Koontz-Lowman D & McKeever-Murphy S (eds), *The Educators Guide to Feeding Children with Disabilities,* Brookes Publishing, Baltimore, MD.

Moore MC & Greene HL, 1985, 'Tube feeding infants and children', *Pediatric Clinics of North America* 32, pp401–17.

Morell P, 1994, 'Low birth weight babies at school age', *Northern neonatal Journal* 2, pp14–48.

Neal P, 1995, 'Special Needs for Special Infants', *Professional Care of Mother and Child* 5 (6) pp151–5.

Nelson CA & Benabib RM, 1991, 'Sensory Preparation in the Oral Motor area', Langley MB & Lambardino L (eds), *Neuro-developmental strategies for Managing Communication Disorders in Children with Severe Motor Dysfunction,* pp131–58, Pro-Ed, Austin, TX.

Norton B, Homer-Ward M, Donnelly MT, Long RG & Holmes GKT, 1996, 'A randomised prospective comparison of percutaneous endoscopic gastrostomy and naso-gastric tube feeding after acute dysphagic stroke', *British Medical Journal* 312, pp13–16.

Ottenbacher K, Scoggins A & Wayland J, 1981, 'The effectiveness of oral sensory motor therapy with the severely and profoundly developmentally disabled', *Occupational Therapy Journal of Research* 1, pp147–60.

Ottenbacher K, Bundy A & Short MA, 1983, The development and treatment of oral-motor dysfunction: a review of clinical research', *Physical and Occupational Therapy in Pediatrics* 3, pp1–13.

Overland L, 2001, Published in advance for Directors in Rehabilitation Magazine (web address www.talktoolstm.com).

Palmer S & Horn S, 1978, 'Feeding Problems in Children', Palmer S & Ekvall S (eds), *Pediatric Nutrition in Developmental Disorders,* Charles C Thomas, Springfield, IL.

Patrick J, Boland M, Stodki D & Murray GE, 1986, 'Rapid correction of wasting in children with Cerebral Palsy', *Developmental Medicine and Child Neurology* 28, pp734–9.

Perske R, Clifton A, McLean BM & Stein JI, 1997, *Mealtimes for severely and profoundly handicapped persons: New concepts and attitudes,* University Park Press, Baltimore, MD.

Randall J, Masalsky CJ & Luiselli JK, 2002, 'Behavioural intervention to increase oral food consumption in an adult with multiple disability and gastrostomy food supplementation', *Journal of Intellectual and Developmental Disability* 27 (1), pp5–13.

Reilly S, 1993, 'Feeding problems in children with cerebral palsy', *Current Paediatrics* 3, pp209–13.

Reilly S & Skuse D, 1992, 'Characteristics and management of feeding problems of young children with cerebral palsy', *Developmental Medicine and Child Neurology* 34, pp379–88.

Reilly S, Skuse D & Poblete X, 1996, 'Prevalence of feeding problems and oral motor dysfunction in children with cerebral palsy – A community survey', *Journal of Pediatrics* 129, pp877–82.

Rempel GR, Colwell SO & Nelson RP, 1998, 'Growth in children with cerebral palsy fed via gastrostomy', *Pediatrics* 82, pp857–62.

Reyes AL, Cash AJ, Green SH & Booth IW, 1993, 'Gastro-oesophageal reflux in children with cerebral palsy', *Child: Care, Health and Development* 19, pp109–18.

Rice H, Seashore JH & Touloukian RJ, 1991, 'Elevation of Nissen fundoplication in neurologically impaired children', *Journal of Pediatric Surgery* 26, pp697–701.

Riordan MM, Iwata BA, Wohl MK & Finney JW, 1980, 'Behavioural Treatment of Food Refusal and Selectivity in Developmentally Disabled Children', *Applied Research in Mental Retardation* 1, pp95–112.

Rogers B, 2004, 'Feeding method and health outcomes of children with cerebral palsy', *Journal of Pediatrics* 145 (2 Suppl), pp28–32.

Rosenfeld-Johnson S, 2001, *Oral-Motor Exercises for Speech Clarity*, Innovative Therapists International, Tucson, AZ.

Shapiro BK, Green P, Krick J, Allen D & Capute AJ, 1986, 'Growth of severely impaired children: Neurological versus nutritional factors, *Developmental Medicine and Child Neurology* 28, pp729–33.

Shellato PC & Malt RA, 1985, 'Tube gastrostomy techniques and complications', *Annals of Surgery* 6, pp180–5.

Shiao SY, Youngblut JM, Anderson GC, DiFiore JM & Martin RJ, 1995, 'Naso-gastric tube placement: effects on breathing and sucking in very-low-birth-weight infants', *Nursing Research* 44 (2), pp82–88.

Sondheimer JM, & Morris BA, 1979, 'Gastro-oesophageal reflux among severely retarded children', *Journal of Pediatrics* 94, pp710–14.

Stallings VA, Charney EB, Davies JC & Cronk CE, 1993, 'Nutrition-related growth failure in children with quadriplegic cerebral palsy', *Developmental Medicine and Child Neurology* 35, pp126–38.

Stevenson RD & Allaire JH, 1996, 'The Development of Eating Skills in Infants and Young Children', pp11–22, Sullivan PB & Rosenbloom L (eds), *Feeding The Disabled Child*, MacKeith Press, London.

Stock Kranowitz C, 1998, *The out of sync child has fun: Activities for kids with sensory integration dysfunction*, The Berkley Publishing Group, NY.

Sullivan PB & Rosenbloom L, 1996, 'The causes of feeding difficulties in disabled children', Sullivan PB & Rosenbloom L (Eds), *Feeding the Disabled Child*, pp23–32, MacKeith Press, London.

Sullivan PB, Lambert B, Rose M, Ford-Adams M, Johnson A, & Griffiths P, 2000, 'Prevalance and Severity of Feeding and nutritional problems in children with neurological impairment: Oxford Feeding Study', *Development Medicine & Child Neurology* 42: pp674–80.

Thomessen M, Kase BF, Riis G & Heiberg A, 1991, 'The impact of feeding problems on growth and energy intake in children with cerebral palsy', *European Journal of Clinical Nutrition* 45, pp479–87.

Troughton KEV & Hill AE, 2001, 'Relationship between objectively measured feeding competence and nutrition in children with cerebral palsy', *Developmental Medicine and Child Neurology* 43, pp187–90.

Vandenberg B & Kielhofner G, 1982, 'Play in Evolution, Culture and Individual Adaptation: Implications for Theory', *American Journal of Occupational Therapy* 36, pp20–28.

Walter RS, 1994, 'Issues surrounding the development of feeding and swallowing', Tuchman DN & Walter RS (eds), *Disorders of Feeding & Swallowing in Children,* pp27–36, Singular, SanDiego, CA.

Wesley JR, Coran G, Sarahan TM, Klein MD & White, SJ, 1993, 'The need for evaluation of gastro-oesophageal reflux associated with severe mental retardation', *Archives of Disease in Childhood* 68, pp347–51.

Wilbarger P, 1995, 'The sensory diet: Activity programs based on sensory processing theory', *Sensory Integration Special Interest Section Newsletter*, 18, pp1–4.

Wilbarger P & Wilbarger J, 2001, *Sensory Defensiveness: A Comprehensive Treatment Approach,* Avanti Educational Programs, Santa Barbara, CA.

Winstock A, 1994, *The Practical Management of Eating & Drinking Difficulties in Children,* Speechmark Publishing, Bicester.

Wolf LS & Glass RP, 1992, *Feeding & Swallowing Disorders in Infancy: Assessment & Management,* Therapy Skill Builders, Tucson, AZ.

Yack E, Sutton S & Aquilla P, 1998, *Building Bridges Through Sensory Integration,* Print 3, Ontario, Canada.

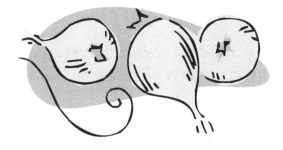

Tools & Resources

NUK® brushes are manufactured by Gerber, PO Box 120, Reedsburg, WI 53959-0120 (www.gerber.com).

Chewy Tubes are manufactured by Speech Pathology Associates, LLC. PO Box 2289, South Portland, ME, 04116 (www.chewytubes.com).

Infadent finger brushes are manufactured by Bolton Dental Manufacturer (BDM) (www.bdmcan.com).

Toothettes were developed by Sage Products Inc (www.sageproducts.com).

Boardmaker is a programme developed by Mayer-Johnson, Inc., PO Box 1579, Solana Beach, CA 92075.

Theraband™ is available from Physio Supplies Limited (www.physiosupplies.com) and ActiveForever.com (www.ActiveForever.com).

Equipment

Sensory oral motor tools and materials can be obtained from companies such as:

Innovative Therapists International (ITI), 3434 E Kleindale Road, Suite F, Tucson, AZ 85716 (website: www.talktoolstm.com).

PDP Products, 14398 North 59th Street, Oak Park Heights, MN 55082 (website: www.pdppro.com).

Super Duper Publications, PO Box 24997, Greenville, SC 29616-2497 (website: www.superduperinc.com).

Speech Dynamics, Inc, 41715 Enterprise Circle N, 107 Temecula, CA 92590 (website: www.speechdynamics.com).

Programmes based on sensory processing theory. *Sensory Integration Special Interest Section Newsletter* 18, pp1–4.

Videos

'Normal Oral Motor & Swallowing Development: Birth to 36 months', Imaginart (available from Winslow Press).

Channel 4 'Life Before Birth', aired April 2005 (www.channel4.com).

Reality Bites: 'Baby it's You'. A Wall to Wall TV production for Channel 4.

Books

Mr Tongue storybook available from www.speechlang.co.uk

Mouth Madness: Oral Motor Activities for Children, Catherine Orr, The Psychological Corporation, USA, 1998.

For Product Safety Concerns and Information please contact our EU
representative GPSR@taylorandfrancis.com Taylor & Francis Verlag GmbH,
Kaufingerstraße 24, 80331 München, Germany

Printed and bound by CPI Group (UK) Ltd, Croydon, CR0 4YY

08/06/2025

01896981-0012